2nd edition

THE ACUTE ABDOMEN

AN APPROACH TO DIAGNOSIS AND MANAGEMENT

THOMAS W. BOTSFORD, M.D., F.A.C.S.

Surgeon, Peter Bent Brigham Hospital
Professor Emeritus, Harvard Medical School

RICHARD E. WILSON, M.D., F.A.C.S.

Surgeon, Peter Bent Brigham Hospital
and Sidney Farber Cancer Institute
Professor of Surgery, Harvard Medical School

W. B. SAUNDERS COMPANY
PHILADELPHIA, LONDON, TORONTO

W. B. Saunders Company: West Washington Square
Philadelphia, PA 19105

1 St. Anne's Road
Eastbourne, East Sussex BN21 3UN, England

1 Goldthorne Avenue
Toronto, Ontario M8Z 5T9, Canada

Listed here is the latest translated edition of this book together
with the language of the translation and the publisher.

Spanish (1st Edition) — Editorial Cientifico-Medica,
Barcelona, Spain

The Acute Abdomen   ISBN   0-7216-1886-3

Print No.:   9   8   7   6   5   4   3   2

It is necessary to begin with the most important things and those most easily recognized. It is necessary to study all that one can see, feel, and hear, everything that one can recognize and use.

HIPPOCRATES, Aphorisms

FOREWORD

A patient with urgent disease in the abdominal cavity is of acute interest to the surgeon as well as to the student and the resident. The patient himself enthusiastically shares this desire for rapid solution of a painful and dangerous crisis in his life. The acute abdomen is a constant challenge, an ever-changing kaleidoscope of pathology, and a happy hunting ground for modern diagnostic techniques; it represents an important fraction of all diagnostic emergencies in medicine, surgery, and pediatrics. In this book, Doctor Botsford and Doctor Wilson have set forth an effective and readable view of the pathologic conditions, the clinical approaches, and the new procedures used to reach that degree of diagnostic certainty essential to treatment.

Our understanding of the nature of the pathologic processes that occur in the human abdomen has not changed in the past 25 years, although its emphasis has. We now see more patients with acute ruptured aneurysms or other vascular accidents (including ischemic enteritis) than we formerly did. This may be because these conditions are commoner in our aging population, or it may reflect the increased interest of the practitioner in trying to rescue some of these older people from vascular calamity. In addition, several complications of new medical and surgical treatments present as cases of acute abdominal pain that were unheard of a decade or two ago. These include such things as small emboli from prosthetic cardiac valves, hemorrhage in patients taking anticoagulants, or acute hepatitis after transfusion.

There has been a marked increase in the range of diagnostic procedures that can be brought to bear. Many are radiologic, including the emergency use of special contrast studies of the gastrointestinal tract, the urinary tract, or the vascular system by angiography or venography. Other new diagnostic procedures, much more widely used now than they were 10 years ago, include diagnostic abdominal paracentesis, emergency blood-enzyme determinations, and isotopic studies.

The greatest advances in the management of patients with acute abdominal conditions have thus come, not from redefinition of the processes that occur, but from the use of new diagnostic procedures. Although the history, the physical examination, and the familiar laboratory work remain the foundation of sound diagnosis and treatment, there has been built upon this ancient base an edifice of refined diagnostic procedures whose use must occupy the attention of every surgeon and student.

Supportive care has also evolved. During the interval between admission and operation, the patient is cared for more effectively than he formerly was. Antibiotics, infusion of fluids and blood, and physiologic support improve the likelihood of survival. This improvement is most noteworthy in the acute abdominal vascular catastrophes. And yet, even with these aids, the mortality from acute abdominal vascular emergencies is still quite high; the keys to improvement in the success rate are to be found in prompt diagnosis, good supportive therapy, and immediate operation.

The authors also emphasize a point that is often over-looked: That a very "acute" abdomen may present itself in a patient who feels quite well and who has very few signs or symptoms of illness. The patient with the acute abdomen is not *always* acutely ill. After blunt trauma to the abdomen in a football game, for example, the patient with the slightest suspicion of left upper quadrant or shoulder pain may be harboring a delayed rupture of the spleen that will endanger his life a few hours or days later. The patient with early intestinal obstruction due to regional enteritis may be almost totally free of pain or dis-comfort when his intestine is empty. And yet, in either case, an acute decision must be made for treatment that is acutely needed.

Hence the acute abdomen and this wonderful book. I know this volume will find a firm place in every hospital library, and in the libraries of many practicing physicians, pediatricians, surgeons, and students of surgery and medicine.

FRANCIS D. MOORE, M.D.

Moseley Professor of Surgery
Harvard Medical School
Surgeon-in Chief
Peter Bent Brigham Hospital

PREFACE
to the Second Edition

In the second edition of this book we have again avoided the nosologic approach to the acute abdomen. Extensive updating and many additions have been made, including chapters on Angiography and Ultrasound. We have not attempted to provide a "cookbook approach" to the care of patients with acute abdominal disease. Rather, it is anticipated that this text will function as a guide for the medical student, intern or resident, and practitioner to learn about and evaluate such patients. Patients suffering from any of the surgical or medical problems described in the book, or even strongly suspected of having them, usually should be under close observation in an emergency room or a hospital until the diagnosis has been proved or dismissed. We have supplied a conceptual framework within which the physician can map a course of action; the decisions and timing must be the individual's.

It is hoped that the new format will lend itself to easy reference in the hospital, the practitioner's office, and the emergency room.

We are indebted to Leroy D. Vandam, M.D., for revising the chapter on Anesthesia. We again thank Edward H. Smith, M.D., for the chapter on Ultrasound, and David C. Levin, M.D., for the chapter on Angiography. The cooperation, patience, and suggestions of our publishers have been most appreciated.

THOMAS W. BOTSFORD, M.D.

RICHARD E. WILSON, M.D.

PREFACE
to the First Edition

This book has been written to present an organized clinical approach to the patient with the "acute abdomen." Rather than lists of organs that may be involved in acute abdominal disease, the basic pathologic process is emphasized. The lesions that may be the cause of the pathologic condition are then developed in relation to it. Actually, experienced clinicians have consciously or unconsciously used this approach for many years. For example, if the patient has an inflammatory disease in his or her abdomen, one starts to sort out the possible causes or organs involved. The same holds true for obstruction, hemorrhage, perforation of a hollow viscus, and abdominal trauma.

A standard diagram of the abdomen, with modification to show the particular lesion or lesions, is used throughout the book. It is hoped that these diagrams will serve as a visual summary of many important points and remind the reader of the many disease conditions that may exist within the peritoneal cavity. A bibliography is purposely not included, but a selected list of references is appended. An extensive bibliography can, paradoxically, detract from a short book such as this.

Finally, it is anticipated that this monograph will function as a guide for the medical student, intern, and resident. Even more important, the practitioner and internist may find it a practical reference, since they frequently are the first to be consulted by the patient with acute abdominal disease.

We again thank Leroy D. Vandam, M.D., for the chapter on Anesthesia and Norman Sadowsky, M.D., for the chapter on Radiology. We are further indebted to Francis D. Moore, M.D., for his invaluable advice and for preparing the Foreword. Mr. Sidney J. Rosenthal was most helpful in designing the overlays on the anatomic diagrams. We are grateful to Mrs. Katharine G. MacDonald for typing the manuscript.

The patience and cooperation of our publishers have been most appreciated.

THOMAS W. BOTSFORD, M.D.

RICHARD E. WILSON, M.D.

BOSTON, MASSACHUSETTS

CONTENTS

SECTION 1   THE TOOLS

SECTION 2   ABDOMINAL TRAUMA

SECTION 3 ACUTE ABDOMINAL INFLAMMATORY DISEASE

SECTION 4 INTESTINAL OBSTRUCTION

SECTION 5   HEMORRHAGE AS A CAUSE OF THE ACUTE ABDOMEN

SECTION 6   THE POSTOPERATIVE ABDOMEN

THE TOOLS

SECTION 1

THE CLINICAL APPROACH TO THE ACUTE ABDOMEN

1

The "acute abdomen" is one of the most common and exciting clinical syndromes encountered in the practice of medicine. At the same time the term "acute abdomen" requires sharp definition. It has been loosely defined as "medical slang for any acute condition within the abdomen demanding immediate operation" (Dorland). A more elegant and succinct definition is: "the acute abdomen is one that requires an acute decision" (F. D. Moore). The decision that invariably and rather quickly must be made is: should or should not the patient be operated upon? If so, how soon?

The patient with an acute abdomen has complaints of brief duration and unknown cause that must be properly diagnosed and treated to prevent mortality or severe morbidity. While the signs or symptoms may be very acute, the underlying lesion may be anything but acute.

In the past, great emphasis has been placed on the accurate diagnosis of the acute abdomen. This ideal is irrefutable, but in reality the exact diagnosis may not be made until an operation is performed, and at times the exact cause of the acute abdomen is not clear even then. The multitude of diseases that can cause an acute abdomen usually present signs or symptoms that fall into one or more of the following four categories: inflammation, with or without perforation of a hollow viscus; obstruction of a hollow viscus; gastrointestinal hemorrhage; and penetrating or blunt abdominal trauma. A working diagnosis that places the patient's problem in one of these categories is often more useful than a "snap diagnosis" or a guess. Moreover, the patient will be more apt to receive proper preoperative preparation and treatment.

In this book a basic anatomic sketch is followed throughout to illustrate the various diagnostic aspects of the acute abdomen. The overall diagram is the same, but the individual points of interest are overlaid on the sketch. For example, in Figure 1-1 the general categories of acute surgical abdominal disease are indicated. It is hoped that this basic sketch with superimposed information will favor continuity of thought on the problem of the acute abdomen and serve to remind the reader that there are many structures in the peritoneal cavity that may be secondarily involved with the primary lesion.

THE TIMING

There are only a few instances of the "acute abdomen" in which minutes count and a delay in operation will produce a fatality. These mostly involve massive hemorrhage from ruptured aortic aneurysm, bullet or stab wounds of the aorta or its major branches or of the

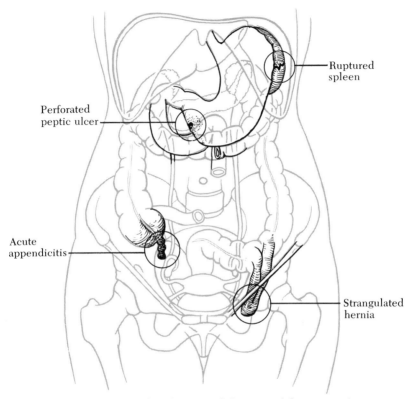

Perforated
peptic ulcer

Ruptured
spleen

Acute
appendicitis

Strangulated
hernia

FIGURE 1–1 Examples of causes of the acute abdomen: sepsis, perforation of a hollow viscus, trauma with hemorrhage, and intestinal obstruction with or without tissue necrosis.

major veins of the abdomen, ruptured spleen, or ruptured ectopic pregnancy. It is mandatory that the hemorrhage be controlled immediately.

There are many conditions that cause the "acute abdomen" in which hours count. In these a delay in operation for some hours significantly increases the morbidity and mortality. They are mostly due to perforation, as in perforation of a duodenal or gastric ulcer, rupture of the appendix, perforation of the gallbladder, free perforation of diverticulitis, intussusception in infancy, saddle embolus to the bifurcation of the aorta, embolus to the mesenteric arterial supply, or trauma.

There is a larger group of acute abdominal conditions in which a delay through a 12-hour period significantly changes the mortality rate. These include small bowel obstruction, incarcerated hernia, mesenteric venous thrombosis, mesenteric arterial thrombosis, acute cholecystitis, appendicitis, acute diverticulitis, volvulus, and other diseases that lead to strangulation of the bowel. In this group careful preoperative preparation for a few hours is an important step in the management.

THE HISTORY

The patient with an acute abdomen seeks medical aid because of a specific complaint. In most instances this is some form of abdominal pain of relatively short duration. Vomiting, inability to move the bowels, gastrointestinal bleeding, weakness, or genitourinary symptoms may be present alone or in association with the pain. The clichés about the history and physical examination are not surveyed in detail here, but they must not be forgotten. A well-versed clinician always thoroughly explores the history and the physical examination. The physician must be able to put all questions in simple everyday terms that the patient can understand. While in this text the vernacular is not used in describing the historical approach, the intelligent physician will talk to the patient in terms that he or she can comprehend. The communication between the patient and the physician must be accurate.

ABDOMINAL PAIN

The answers to the following four questions will provide important clues to exactly what has happened and is happening to the patient.

When did the pain start and what was the mode of onset? The answer tells the approximate duration of the pain but not that of the lesion. It must be remembered that the disease may have been present for some time before the pain started. For example, anorexia, apathy, and malaise are usually present prior to the onset of pain from inflammatory lesions. Tumors obviously predate the intestinal obstruction they cause. The mode is important. The explosive violent pain of a perforated hollow viscus or a vascular accident is entirely different from the gradually increasing pain of an inflammatory lesion.

What is the nature of the pain? Is it steady and unrelenting or intermittent and crampy? The pain of inflammatory lesions and peritoneal irritation is steady, whereas that of bowel obstruction or colic is intermittent. What makes it better or worse?

What is the severity of the pain and how rapid was the onset? An excruciating persistent pain not relieved by morphine suggests a vascular lesion such as mesenteric thrombosis or a dissecting aortic aneurysm. An explosive onset associated with collapse is characteristic of a ruptured viscus or vascular accident. A rapidly progressive pain suggests mesenteric thrombosis, acute pancreatitis, or strangulated hernia. Abdominal pain that is slow and gradual in development is more characteristic of inflammatory lesions such as diverticulitis or appendicitis.

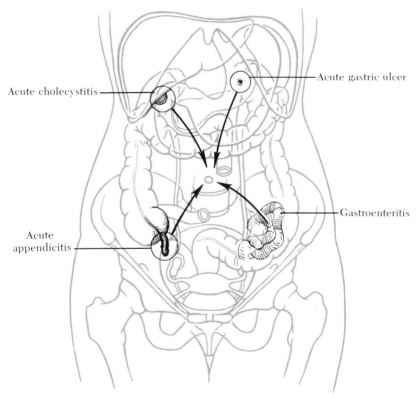

FIGURE 1–2   The initial radiation of pain to upper or mid abdomen in several acute abdominal diseases.

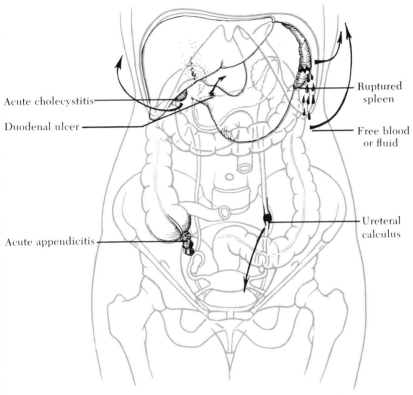

Acute cholecystitis

Duodenal ulcer

Ruptured spleen

Free blood or fluid

Ureteral calculus

Acute appendicitis

FIGURE 1–3 Other patterns of radiation of pain caused by acute cholecystitis, appendicitis, peptic ulcer, ruptured spleen, and ureteral calculus. Pain from appendicitis localizes in the right lower quadrant.

Where is the pain located and did it radiate? It is most helpful to obtain a fairly discrete idea of where the pain started and to note the radiation. Figures 1-2 and 1-3 show the localization of some pain areas and radiation.

VOMITING

Vomiting is such a ubiquitous act that it can be clarified in simple terms. Vomiting without pain or that has preceded the pain by a considerable period of time probably is not associated with a surgical lesion. The presence or absence of gross or occult blood in the vomitus is of obvious significance. The presence of bile in the vomitus means that there is no pyloric obstruction. Persistent vomiting soon after the onset of pain suggests high intestinal obstruction. Vomiting first of food and gastric contents, then bile, and finally feculent material indicates low intestinal obstruction. Repeated vomiting and persistent nausea are common in acute pancreatitis. Spontaneous vomiting associated with right upper quadrant or right lower quadrant pain is characteristic of acute cholecystitis and appendicitis. If the vomiting brings relief of pain, it suggests an obstructive lesion with temporary decompression.

GASTROINTESTINAL BLEEDING

With massive bleeding from the esophagus, stomach, or duodenum, the patient may vomit bright red blood mixed with clots. If the bleeding is at a slower rate, the vomitus will look like "coffee grounds." Bleeding from the upper jejunum may first be apparent in vomitus rather than as melena. In other words, vomiting of blood does not rule out the possibility of an upper small bowel lesion.

Bleeding from the rectum may vary from the streak of bright blood associated with a fissure-in-ano or hem-

orrhoid to the tarry stool of upper gastrointestinal hemorrhage. In general, bright red blood by rectum indicates a
low-lying cause; however, the color of the blood passed
may be misleading. If the rate of bleeding is rapid and
peristalsis is active, blood from a point high in the intestine may be passed by the rectum relatively unchanged.

TRAUMA

The details of the accident, if available, are important
in the appraisal of the extent of injury. The history may
not be obtainable or may be a single phrase such as "car
accident," "stab wound," or "gunshot wound." The primary considerations in the life of the patient and the examination cannot be dissociated from the management.
The priorities are to provide an adequate airway,
emergency resuscitation if necessary, and control of obvious serious blood loss. A rapid survey of the extent of the
injuries can be made then, and indicated procedures
carried out.

GUIDES FOR THE PHYSICAL EXAMINATION

1. Usually the patient with an acute abdomen looks
ill. Occasionally, a truly important acute abdominal condition can masquerade in a patient with very few complaints. If the patient is in pain, it is obvious, and he or
she does not appreciate the frequent probing of an area
of tenderness. The patient is apprehensive and irritable
for good reason, being frightened and impatient to be
relieved of the cause of his or her pain.

2. It is wise to defer the painful part of the examination to the end. If done first, the patient will become tense and difficult to examine. For example, listen for peristalsis prior to palpating the abdominal wall.

3. Never omit searching for a strangulated femoral, inguinal, or ventral hernia.

4. Use the right hand as well as the left to do the pelvic examination. A twisted right ovarian cyst can be more easily palpated with the right hand than with the left.

5. Always do a pelvic and rectal examination yourself. Do not accept the findings of others. The findings may have changed by the time you do it.

6. The sign of contralateral tenderness helps to distinguish between thoracic disease that is causing abdominal pain and rigidity and an acute inflammatory process in an upper quadrant of the abdomen. Pressure on the opposite quadrant of the abdomen carried in deeply toward the affected side usually causes pain if the lesion is intraabdominal but does not cause pain if the disease is above the diaphragm.

7. Always palpate the abdomen again after medication for pain has been given. A mass not felt before may be found or a more detailed appraisal of a previously detected mass can be made.

8. Do not hesitate to insert a nasogastric tube if indicated at the end of a physical examination. Valuable knowledge can be obtained from analysis of the gastric contents. The presence or absence of free acid and the character of the gastric contents can provide important diagnostic information. In addition, gastric decompression will begin immediately.

9. In the same fashion, an inlying urethral catheter

is most important in the very ill patient. It should be placed early so that urinary output may be measured accurately.

10. Aspiration of the peritoneal cavity is a valuable diagnostic procedure. Commonly known as the peritoneal "tap," it may provide immediate and decisive information for the care of the patient. It is a rapid method of determining whether there is free blood or pus present in the peritoneal cavity. Thus a positive tap becomes highly significant, but a negative tap does not rule out the presence of intraabdominal disease. The abdominal fluid may be out of reach of the aspirating needle, or improper technique may have been used.

The method is easy and safe to carry out. Peritoneal aspiration should not be attempted at the site of an abdominal scar or over solid abdominal viscera. A suitable syringe (10 to 12 ml.) with a long No. 18-gauge needle is used. The syringe should contain 5 or 10 ml. of saline so that a little can be injected ahead of the needle to make the procedure safer and to provide some irrigation. A wheal of local anesthetic is raised in the skin of the abdominal quadrant to be tapped. The needle is gently inserted through the abdominal wall into the peritoneal cavity. When the peritoneum is penetrated, the patient may have a twinge of pain. Usually it is easy to determine when the peritoneum is entered. The needle need not enter the abdominal cavity more than one-half inch for adequate aspiration. The fluid obtained can be cultured, smeared, and examined chemically if indicated. The tap can be made in any of the quadrants of the abdomen (Figure 1–4); at times multiple taps may be indicated. Its chief value is in the patient who has suffered blunt abdominal trauma. Like that of many other an-

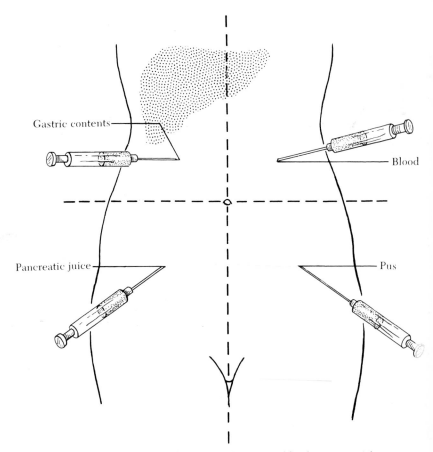

FIGURE 1–4 Four-quadrant tap. Free pus, blood, or material from a perforated viscus may be obtained for diagnostic study.

cillary maneuvers, the result, especially if negative, does not replace the clinical indication or the desirability of a necessary surgical operation.

11. While the four quadrant abdominal tap is quick and simple to perform, diagnostic peritoneal lavage may help in those patients who have suffered blunt trauma with multiple injuries and uncertain physical findings. A small infraumbilical incision is made under local anesthesia (after the urinary bladder is emptied) and an intravenous plastic catheter is carefully inserted into the peritoneal cavity. If blood or intestinal contents are obtained, the procedure is terminated as a positive test. Otherwise, 1 liter of sterile balanced saline solution is instilled into the peritoneal cavity and then aspirated. The fluid is examined grossly and microscopically, and chemical tests (such as the amylase content) can be performed on it as indicated.

LAPAROSCOPY IN ACUTE ABDOMINAL CONDITIONS

Laparoscopy or peritoneoscopy is gaining wide acceptance as a diagnostic technique. The development of more sophisticated fiber-optic lighting systems and the broad application of the laparoscope in a variety of surgical fields have led to its increasing use in patients with acute abdominal complaints. Laparoscopy is a procedure with low risk and may greatly increase the accuracy of preoperative diagnosis in this type of patient. Laparoscopy can be performed under local anesthesia and may find its greatest usefulness in separating those patients who have acute abdominal conditions requiring early surgery from those who do not. Unnecessary procedures may be avoided in patients with superficial stab wounds, pancreatitis, pelvic inflammatory disease, and acute duodenal ulcer. On the other hand, its use may speed the decision for surgery in patients with appendicitis, ectopic pregnancy, or ruptured spleen. In this regard, a review of the use of laparoscopy at the Peter Bent Brigham Hospital as an aid in the diagnosis of acute abdominal pain demonstrated a significant reduction in cost of hospital care for patients so studied.

The laparoscope is introduced through a small subumbilical incision and the abdomen is examined after the peritoneal cavity is distended with CO_2. The patient's urinary bladder should be emptied before the instrument is inserted, and the instrument should not be inserted through an abdominal scar. Introduction of a probe through a counter incision can greatly increase the ability of the operator to visualize more of the peritoneal contents. The more experienced surgeons become with its use in the diagnosis of the acute abdomen, the longer will be the list of disease states that can be determined and followed by laparoscopic techniques.

LABORATORY AIDS IN DIAGNOSIS OF THE ACUTE ABDOMEN

2

A tremendous array of sophisticated laboratory aids exists to help the clinician arrive at more accurate diagnoses and better therapy. Despite this, the commonplace white blood cell count, blood smear, hematocrit, urinalysis, and examination of the stool for blood are sharp tools in the diagnosis of the acute abdomen. In acute abdominal disease, a working diagnosis must be made rather quickly, so that time limits the feasibility of many laboratory tests. It is, therefore, important that the clinician caring for the patient make maximum use of those laboratory tests that are immediately available. It also must be remembered that laboratory tests are not substitutes for clinical astuteness. Ambiguities may exist in laboratory studies, and occasional errors and inaccuracies make them no better than the individual or instrument that performed them.

Throughout this book, specific laboratory studies that may be of great diagnostic usefulness in certain problems are mentioned. In this section an attempt is made to provide a background of the various laboratory studies that are available. Many of them apply more to the care of the sick patient than to the initial diagnosis of the disease. For the purpose of completeness, a table of

TABLE 2–1   Normal Chemical Values in Blood

Determination	Minimum Volume Whole Blood	Normal Range
Amylase	3 ml.	40–120 Somogyi units
Bilirubin, total	3 ml.	0.1–1.0 mg./100 ml.
Bilirubin, direct	3 ml.	0.1–0.3 mg./100 ml.
BSP retention	3 ml.	Less than 8% in 45 min.
Calcium	3 ml.	4.4–5.6 mEq./L.
Chloride	3 ml.	99–111 mEq./L.
CO_2 combining power	3 ml.	22–30 mM/L.
CO_2 content	3 ml.	22–30 mM/L.
Creatinine*	3 ml.	0.7–1.3 mg./100 ml. (male)
		0.5–1.0 mg./100 ml. (female)
Creatine phosphokinase (CPK)	4 ml.	0–12 sigma units
Glutamic oxaloacetic transaminase (GOT)	4 ml.	11–33 Henry units
Lactic dehydrogenase (LDH)	3 ml.	131–231 Wacker units
Lipase	8 ml.	0–1 units
Oxygen saturation, arterial blood	3 ml.	96–100%
pH, arterial blood	3 ml.	7.35–7.45
Phosphatase, alkaline	2 ml.	9–41 I.U.
Phosphorus	3 ml.	0.9–1.5 mM/L.
Potassium	3 ml.	3.8–5.0 mEq./L.
Albumin	3 ml.	4.0–5.6 gm./100 ml.
Protein, total	3 ml.	6.3–7.9 gm./100 ml.
Sodium	3 ml.	138–144 mEq./L.
Sugar*	3 ml.	75–120 mg./100 ml.
Urea*	3 ml.	8–25 mg./100 ml.
Uric acid	3 ml.	3.7–7.5 mg./100 ml. (male)
		2.8–5.8 mg./100 ml. (female)

*Indicates that the analysis may be done on serum or plasma. All other blood analyses are carried out on serum only.

normal values obtained by standard laboratory tests is included (Table 2–1).

BLOOD STUDIES

WHITE BLOOD CELL COUNT

The white blood cell count assumes primary importance in the diagnosis of the acute abdomen. The total count is usually elevated and is highly significant, but at times in acute disease sufficient time has not elapsed for the elevation to occur. This may be true even in certain situations such as appendicitis, perforated peptic ulcer, massive hemorrhage, and trauma. Repeated observations of white blood cell counts showing gradual elevation over a period of time may become significant in making a diagnosis in borderline situations like early appendicitis. However, the white blood cell count, regardless of its level, does not supersede the clinical evidence of the disease. Rather, the white cell count will strengthen the diagnostic impression, not void it. In general, the leukocyte count is increased in inflammatory disease of the abdomen, and a progressively rising count over a period of hours or days is strong evidence of active infection. In common acute gastroenteritis, the leukocyte count is usually not elevated, nor is it in mesenteric adenitis. A leukopenia may exist in certain conditions, and the inordinately low white blood cell count may provide a clue to the diagnosis. Such diseases include typhoid fever, gram-negative sepsis, some of the leukemias, and pernicious anemia and other pancytopenias.

BLOOD SMEAR

The examination of the blood smear, particularly the differential count of the white blood cells, may be most helpful. Generally polymorphonuclear leukocytes are present in increased numbers in any inflammatory reaction, and the presence of band forms is an even greater indication of reaction to inflammation. In the very young and the very old, the white blood cell count may be misleading as these age groups often do not react normally to infection. Stippling of the leukocytes (toxic reaction) may be associated with severe or overwhelming infections.

The eosinophil count may be helpful in detecting parasitic infestation and allergic reactions. It is increased in both instances. An absolute increase in lymphocytes may be associated with adrenal cortical insufficiency, which may evoke vomiting, abdominal pain, and fever. Abnormal lymphocytes in the smear may be the first clue to infectious mononucleosis, lymphoma, or leukemia.

Basophilic stippling of the erythrocytes, particularly if accompanied by the blue line of the gums, may lead to the diagnosis of colic associated with lead poisoning. The sickle cells of the anemia of that name cannot be seen in the routine smear but are demonstrated in wet preparation.

HEMATOCRIT AND ERYTHROCYTE COUNT

In dealing with the acute abdomen, the hematocrit is preferable to the red blood cell count. It can be done easily with greater accuracy and more reproducible results, and will more effectively detect changes in plasma volume. It can, however, be misleading in instances of acute or chronic blood loss. During acute bleeding and immediate blood transfusions, it tends to remain normal. In more chronic bleeding, transcapillary refilling occurs and further dilution of the already reduced number of red blood cells falsely lowers the hematocrit.

It is most important, therefore, that the hematocrit not be used as the single guide to blood volume or the imminence of shock, or to determine whether or not active bleeding is continuing in any given patient. The vital signs of the blood pressure, pulse, and respiration and the patient's general appearance are of far greater value here than the hematocrit. The hematocrit is much more effective and more rapidly discloses changes in plasma volume than changes in the red cell volume. Lesions such as burns, pancreatitis, peritonitis, superior mesenteric vascular occlusion, and strangulation of the bowel are associated with a rise in the hematocrit and concomitant fall in the circulating plasma volume. By making use of the hematocrit and an estimate of the patient's weight, the patient's normal blood volume can be estimated. Then a fairly close approximation of the plasma loss can be made by using the ratio of the normal to the abnormal hematocrit (Table 2–2).

The hematocrit may be of value in other ways. An unexplained or unsuspected anemia, as shown by a low hematocrit, may point toward a lesion causing chronic blood loss; the lesion now is the cause of acute abdominal signs and symptoms. Examples are sudden obstruction or perforation of a carcinoma or peptic ulcer. Gastric aspiration may detect the site of the blood loss. Likewise, sigmoidoscopy may demonstrate the colonic

TABLE 2–2   Calculation of Plasma Volume Deficit*

$$PV\ deficit = BV_1 - \frac{(BV_1 \times LVH_1)}{LVH_2}$$

PV = plasma volume

when: BV_1 = normal blood volume for the patient as estimated from body weight, build, and sex
(adult male—7% B.W.)
(adult female—6.5% B.W.)

LVH_1 = normal large vessel hematocrit for this individual (expressed as a decimal)

LVH_2 = observed LVH (expressed as a decimal)

Example: An 80-kg. man with acute pancreatitis enters the hospital with a hematocrit of 58%. Normal hematocrit may be estimated at 40%.

BV_1 = 5600 ml.

$$PV\ deficit = 5600 - \frac{(5600 \times 0.40)}{0.58}$$

PV deficit = 5600 − 3860

PV deficit = 1740 ml.

*Adapted from Moore, F. D.: Metabolic Care of the Surgical Patient. Philadelphia, W. B. Saunders Company, 1959, p. 217.

tumor that has been insidiously bleeding and is now the cause of large bowel obstruction.

PLATELET COUNT

The platelet count occasionally may be helpful in acute abdominal problems. Petechiae associated with a low platelet count may provide a clue to the cause of intraluminal bleeding or to a lesion such as splenic infarct as a cause of retroperitoneal bleeding. Intraabdominal sepsis due to gram-negative organisms may be associated with thrombocytopenia.

SERUM ELECTROLYTES

The serum electrolyte values may not be of any great usefulness in the diagnosis of problems of the acute abdomen, but they will be exceedingly important in the preparation of the patient for operation and his or her postoperative care. Since many acute abdominal conditions produce widespread tissue injury and complex surgical procedures may be required, predictably, fluid and electrolyte therapy can be complicated. A basic knowledge of the management of fluids and their electrolyte components is essential.

As a basis for fluid and electrolyte therapy and for specific diagnostic problems related to abnormalities in fluid and electrolytes, it is essential that the electrolyte content of the serum and other body fluids be known to the physician; the normal ranges of values for these are seen in Table 2–3. An understanding of the content of

TABLE 2–3   Electrolyte Concentrations in Gastrointestinal Tract Drainage

	Range of Values (mEq./Liter)*				
	Na^+	CL^-	K^+	HCO_3^-	H^+
Gastric fluid					
(high acid)	45–70	110–120	20–35	20–25	70 pH (1.5)
(low acid)	90–100	115–120	40–50	30–35	<1 pH (5.5)
Small intestinal fluid	110–125	100–110	20–40	25–30	
Bile	130–145	100–110†	30–40	30–40	
Pancreatic juice	140–160	70–100†	10–30	25–150	
Colonic and low ileal fluid	110–130	100–110	30–50	25–30	

*These values are meant to serve only as an initial guideline. For patients with continuous extrarenal losses, it is recommended that determinations be made on aliquots of the drainage.

†The chloride concentration is inversely proportional to the bicarbonate level in the drainage.

various intravenous fluids usually used for therapy is necessary as well. Isotonic saline or dextrose and saline contain 155 mEq. of sodium and chloride per liter of fluid. Concentrated 3 per cent sodium chloride solutions contain 55 mEq. per 100 ml. of sodium and chloride. Lactated Ringer's solution contains 130 mEq. of sodium per liter.

There are certain metabolic abnormalities most frequently associated with acute abdominal problems. These include: hypokalemic alkalosis, acute desalting water loss, acute dehydration, acute respiratory acidosis, hypokalemia of chronic constipation, and low-perfusion lactic acidosis. All of these except respiratory acidosis must be suitably treated by fluid and electrolyte therapy, and they play a very significant role in the eventual outcome for the patient with an acute abdomen. Their diagnosis can be arrived at by obtaining serum electrolyte as well as arterial blood gas determinations. The partial pressure of carbon dioxide in the blood (Pco_2) and the oxygen saturation and the partial pressure of oxygen (Po_2) in the blood greatly aid in the management of acutely ill patients. Respiratory complications are a major cause of death in surgical patients; it is the individual with an acute abdominal problem who is most likely to have had poor respiratory preparation and to develop subsequent respiratory difficulties. Knowledge of these arterial blood gas values, coupled with pulmonary function values such as vital capacity, timed vital capacity, and maximum breathing capacity, helps the surgeon decide whether such measures as tracheostomy, positive pressure breathing, oxygen administration, and additional buffering agents are necessary for any given patient. The ability to save the lives of patients with serious acute injuries and illness hinges on the ability to correct deficiencies in these areas.

Serum calcium and phosphate determinations may be helpful in checking for hyperparathyroidism in patients with renal stone disease and in patients with pancreatitis or duodenal ulcer. The soap formation that occurs in acute pancreatitis may actually produce hypocalcemia, and the diagnosis may sometimes be arrived at as a result of this. Abdominal pain due to metastatic malignant disease with back pain may be associated with hypercalcemia, and again, the diagnosis may be aided by this knowledge. Severe ileus may result from abnormalities of calcium, potassium, or phosphate in the serum.

Other serum constituents that should be considered at the same time as electrolytes are the serum bilirubin and the serum proteins, which may be abnormal in patients with liver disease or biliary tract disease and certainly can play a significant role in the diagnosis of these problems.

ENZYMES

The serum amylase determination is certainly a useful and commonly performed test in dealing with the acute abdomen. The LDH (lactic dehydrogenase) may be markedly elevated in sepsis and tissue necrosis. The SGOT (serum glutamic oxaloacetic transaminase) may be indicative of hepatic disease and to some extent reflects tissue injury. A rise in the LDH without a concomitant elevation of the SGOT may be diagnostic of a pulmonary embolism, one of the medical problems occasionally confused with an acute abdomen.

URINALYSIS AND STOOL EXAMINATION

URINALYSIS

The routine urine examination assumes great importance in the acute abdomen. Dilute urine accompanied by severe vomiting may point to renal disease. The significance of blood or white blood cells in the urine is obvious, as is the presence of bile or sugar.

THE STOOL

A specimen of stool is always available from the gloved finger of the examining hand. A test for occult blood can be done rapidly and should not be omitted. A Gram stain of the stool for predominant organisms can be very useful in the debilitated patient or one in whom pseudomembranous colitis is suspected.

ROENTGENOLOGIC EXAMINATION OF THE ACUTE ABDOMEN

*NORMAN L. SADOWSKY, M.D.**

3

Roentgenologic examination of the patient with acute abdominal disease should be considered an extension of the physical examination. It is important that the limitations as well as the usefulness of this diagnostic tool be recognized. For proper interpretation, the films must be technically good and the radiologist must be acquainted with the patient's clinical findings. It is imperative that the surgeon and the radiologist consult with each other in order to obtain the maximum information about these acutely ill patients. Many different terms are used to indicate the roentgenograms of the abdomen made without previous preparation or the introduction of

*Chief, Department of Radiology, Faulkner Hospital, Boston; Associate Professor of Radiology, Tufts Medical School, Boston.

contrast media. Some of these are "scout films," "flat films," "plain films," "KUB," "preliminary films," "pilot films," and "survey films." The term "survey film" is used in this discussion.

INSPECTION OF THE SURVEY FILM

The landmarks of the normal anteroposterior abdominal roentgenogram should be familiar not only to the radiologist but to the physician or surgeon (Figure 3–1). A systematic plan of inspection of the x-ray film should be completely followed. If it is not, much can be lost. For example, dilated loops of small bowel may be seen, but the gallstone causing the obstruction may be missed or the fractured vertebrae with ileus may be overlooked. The following is a plan for looking at the abdominal roentgenograms of the acute abdomen systematically.

SOLID ORGANS

The outline of the liver, spleen, kidneys, and psoas muscle margins should be specifically inspected and note made of the position and size of these organs. Transposition of the viscera is rare but can be recognized by the position of the liver, so that a left-sided cholecystitis could be recognized. Splenomegaly in a bleeding patient may alert one to the possibility of esophageal varices. Poor visualization of the enlarged spleen and an associated rib fracture point to a ruptured spleen. Loss of sharpness of outline of one psoas margin may indicate a

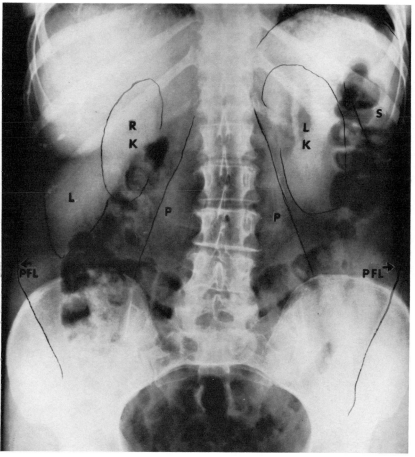

FIGURE 3–1 Normal landmarks and organs can be seen on the survey film of the abdomen. L, liver; RK, right kidney; LK, left kidney; S, tip of spleen; PFL, peritoneal fat lines; P, psoas muscle.

retroperitoneal process (bleeding or inflammation), and absence of the hepatic angle outline indicates free fluid in the abdominal cavity. Enlargement of a kidney sometimes is seen in acute ureteral obstruction. The presence of horseshoe kidney may be the etiology of an abdominal mass. A suprarenal mass may be seen in the plain film as well.

HOLLOW ORGANS

The hollow organs often can be seen quite well because of the gas contained within them. Air or gas normally is seen in the stomach and colon, and small amounts are not unusual in the small bowel. Dilatation of the stomach with air and fluid is seen in obstructing ulcers. Localized dilatation of the small bowel in the region of the ligament of Treitz is often seen in acute pancreatitis (Figures 3-2 and 3-3). The position of the colon and the degree of distention of all or part of it will help in the diagnosis of large bowel obstruction, malrotation, volvulus, ulcerative colitis with toxic dilatation, and appendicitis.

The presence of free air in the abdomen can be detected in an upright film, where it can be seen under the diaphragms (Figure 3-4), or in a lateral decubitus film, rising to the upper side of the abdomen. Free air in the abdomen is indubitable proof of perforation of a hollow viscus; it may be seen up to 6 days following laparotomy and for even longer periods when adhesions or peritonitis is present. Allowing the patient to remain upright or lying on the left side for five minutes prior to taking upright or decubitus films, respectively, will reduce the

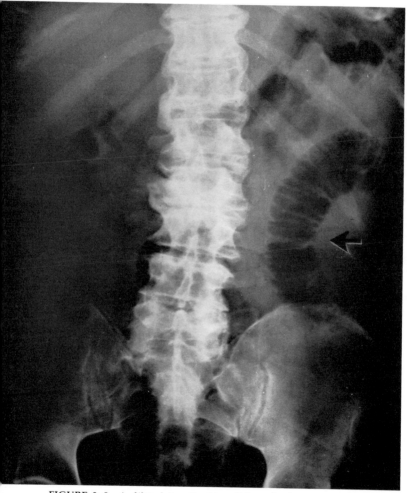

FIGURE 3–2   A dilated "sentinel loop" (*arrow*) of small bowel is often a feature of acute pancreatitis.

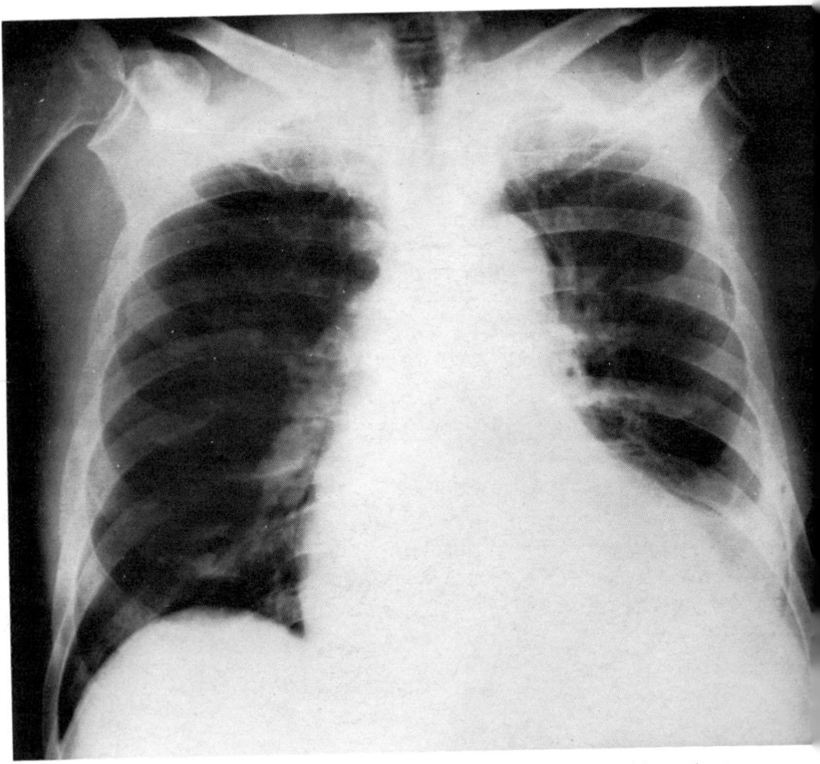

FIGURE 3–3 Left pleural effusion in the same pancreatitis patient as shown in Figure 3–2.

possibility of a false negative examination if a small perforation has occurred. The most common cause of free air in the abdomen is perforation of a peptic ulcer. Air in this case is often best demonstrated with the patient in the left lateral decubitus position, which allows gas to es-

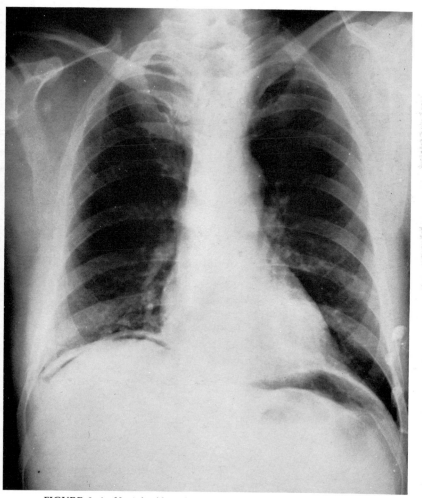

FIGURE 3–4   Upright film of the chest shows free air under both diaphragms. The patient had a perforated duodenal ulcer.

cape from the stomach as it rises to the right side. A large amount of free air may result from colonic perforation, and often the diagnosis can be made in the recumbent film when one sees both the outer and inner walls of the bowel with gas both within and outside the bowel lumen. Since only small amounts of gas are normally present in the small bowel, it is not unusual not to see any free air in the small bowel perforations. Free air is also unusual in appendiceal abscess; occasionally small bubbles may be seen in the region of the cecum or under the liver.

Gas shadows in the liver conforming to the distribution of the biliary tree can be seen in patients with choledochoduodenostomy or cholecystoduodenostomy of either spontaneous or surgical origin. When seen with dilatation of the small bowel, it may indicate gallstone ileus. Gas in the hepatic vascular tree is seen in mesenteric thrombosis, strangulating obstructions, and ulcerating gastrointestinal lesions.

The differentiation between paralytic ileus and intestinal obstruction can often be difficult. Ileus may be seen after operation, cystoscopy, intravenous urography, apprehension, and conscious air swallowing as well as in acute abdominal disease or trauma. The survey film shows gas throughout the small bowel, large bowel, and stomach. Upright films may show air fluid levels in paralytic ileus, but these tend to be long and few rather than the multiple short stepladder levels seen in intestinal obstruction (Figures 3–5 and 3–6). In uncomplicated obstruction, only the bowel proximal to the obstruction is distended, while in ileus the distention is generalized. It is not unusual for paralytic ileus to be superimposed on actual obstruction if the process is prolonged. In low

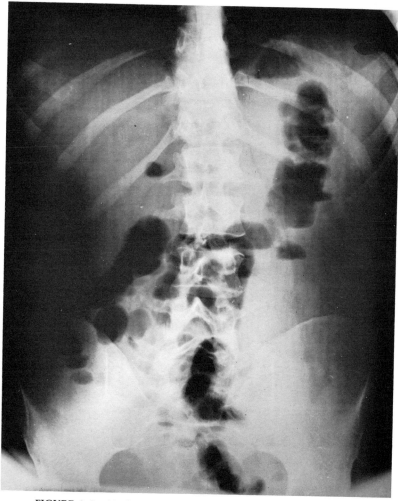

FIGURE 3-5 Air-fluid levels in a patient with small bowel obstruction.

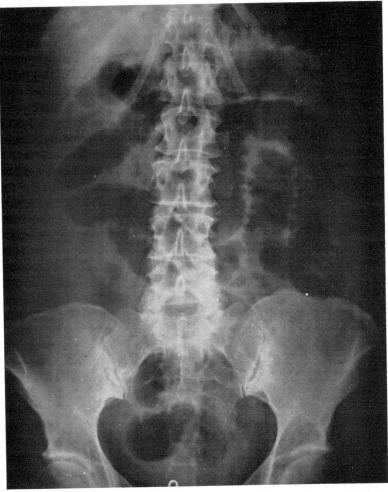

FIGURE 3–6 The bowel is dilated and the valvulae conniventes are visualized in small bowel obstruction.

large bowel obstruction the colon alone may be distended if the ileocecal valve is competent (Figures 3–7 and 3–8). In the absence of a competent ileocecal valve, distal large bowel obstruction may produce a generalized distention that can be distinguished from ileus only after a barium enema shows the obstructing lesion. The splenic flexure cutoff sign (in which gaseous distention abruptly stops at the splenic flexure) may be seen in superior mesenteric artery thrombosis and acute pancreatitis as well as in obstruction due to intrinsic colonic disease. Displacement of the hepatic or splenic flexure may indicate laceration of the liver or spleen. Sigmoid and cecal volvulus present characteristic gas patterns with dilatation of the sigmoid loop in the right upper quadrant in the former and dilatation of the cecum in the left upper quadrant in the latter (Figures 3–9 and 3–10).

The ability to distinguish large from small bowel loops is extremely important, and the distinction is sometimes difficult. The large bowel occupies a position around the periphery of the abdomen while, in general, the small bowel lies within the perimeter thus formed. Another differential point is based on the presence of the three bands of longitudinal muscle (teniae coli) that divide the colonic haustra so that haustral folds cannot be traced in a continuous line across the bowel, while small bowel folds usually can be seen as an uninterrupted line. The colonic sacculations, of course, are quite characterisitc.

The amount of gas and its distribution in the bowel in obstruction depend on the location of the obstruction and the length of time since onset. It may take 6 hours or longer for a sufficient amount of gas to accumulate proximal to the obstruction to enable one to pinpoint its loca-

Text continued on page 42

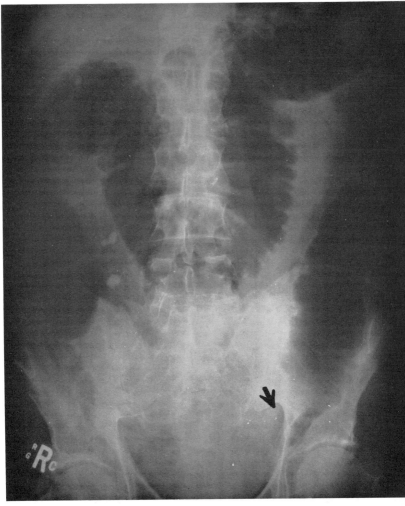

FIGURE 3–7   The large bowel is dilated and the point of obstruction is indicated by the arrow. There is no dilatation of the small bowel, as this patient had a competent ileocecal valve.

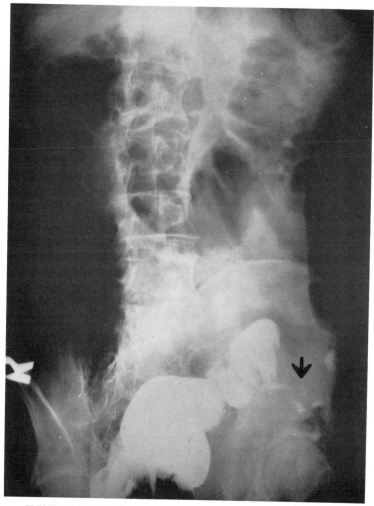

FIGURE 3–8 The barium enema study in the same patient depicted in Figure 3–7. The arrow indicates the site of the obstructing carcinoma. Note the dilated colon proximal to the lesion.

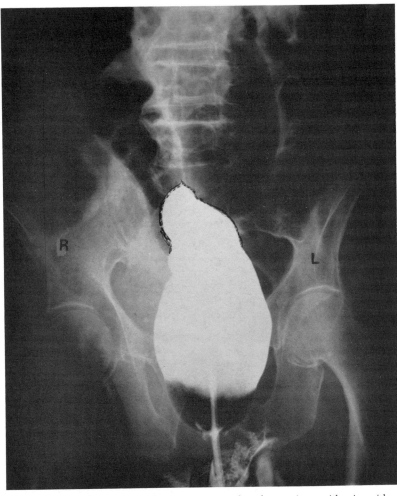

FIGURE 3–9 Barium enema study of a patient with sigmoid volvulus. Note the "bird's beak" deformity at the point where the bowel is twisted.

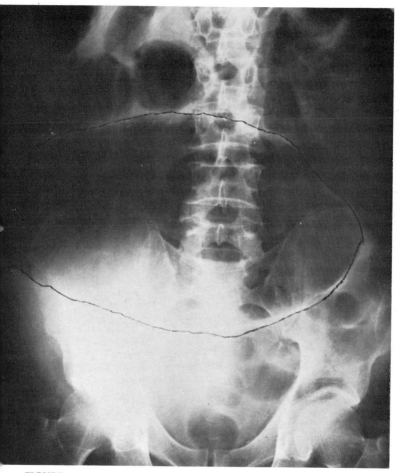

FIGURE 3–10   Volvulus of the cecum. The huge dilated right colon extends into the left side of the abdomen.

tion. Since almost all the gas in the bowel is from ingested air, gas tends to pass out and not reaccumulate in loops distal to an obstruction. In the supine film, however, fluid may accumulate just proximal to the obstruction so that these loops cannot be seen. More valuable than an upright film in locating the point of obstruction is a prone film, since in the upright position fluid tends to flow into the dependent bowel loops. The prone film, on the other hand, causes a shift in distribution of gas and fluid that, together with the appearance on the supine film, may pinpoint the obstruction exactly. The use of barium in small bowel obstruction is discussed later.

BONY STRUCTURES

Inspection of the bony structures (ribs, vertebrae, pelvis, and hips) should be carefully carried out. Fractures of the lower ribs are often associated with splenic rupture or hepatic laceration, and fractures of the transverse processes may be associated with retroperitoneal hemorrhage or renal trauma. A fractured pelvis should point to the possibility of trauma to the bladder, which can be confirmed by a cystogram. Inspection of the symmetry of the hip joints will prevent one from overlooking a posterior dislocation of the hip, which may accompany blunt trauma in motor accidents, and to correct this injury immediately is to prevent aseptic necrosis. Destructive or osteoblastic lesions from metastatic tumor and generalized bone demineralization should also be looked for.

ABDOMINAL SOFT TISSUE MASSES

A large soft tissue mass found in the pelvis may represent a distended bladder. Masses due to ovarian or uterine tumors usually can be distinguished from the bladder in the survey film by virtue of the fine radiolucent fat line between the mass and the collapsed bladder. A large soft tissue pseudotumor projecting into the stomach shadow is sometimes seen in pancreatitis, and another pseudotumor mass can be seen in strangulating obstruction of the small bowel.

CALCIFICATIONS

Calcification normally may be present in bone and costal cartilage with incidental calcification in lymph nodes, spleen, and occasionally liver. Vascular calcification is often seen in the splenic artery, aorta, and iliac and pelvic vessels; these assume importance when thrombosis or aneurysm is considered in the differential diagnosis. One looks for calculi in the biliary tree, urinary system, and pancreas (Figure 3–11). Comparison with previous films can be extremely important in assessing the significance of calculi; any change in size or position should be looked for. The disappearance of a gallstone from the right upper quadrant may alert one to look for gas in the biliary tree and gallstone ileus. Uterine fibroids show gross amorphous calcification as opposed to the spotty calcification in ovarian cystadenomas. Tooth and bone formation in a pelvic mass indicates a dermoid cyst. The presence of a large foreign body in the abdomen may be a valuable clue in the diagnosis of bowel

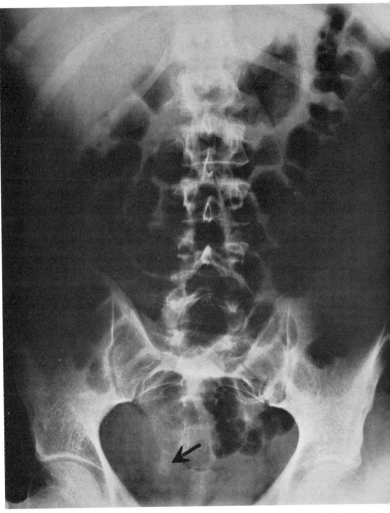

FIGURE 3–11   The scout film shows an area of calcification indicated by the arrow. This calcification proved to be a calcified appendiceal fecalith.

perforation and abscess or intestinal obstruction. Metallic sutures in the abdomen, evidence of previous surgery, may indicate the presence of adhesions.

SPECIAL CONTRAST STUDIES

Special contrast studies such as the barium enema, intravenous urography, intravenous cholangiogram, and upper gastrointestinal series are frequently necessary aids in the diagnosis of the acute abdomen. If indicated, these procedures should be done immediately regardless of the time of day or night. An upper gastrointestinal series using a water-soluble opaque medium may be indicated in cases in which perforation of the duodenum due to peptic ulcer or blunt abdominal trauma is suspected. Oral barium can be very helpful in the diagnosis of splenic rupture since it can show any displacement of the greater curvature of the stomach by the enlarging splenic mass; a left lateral decubitus film as well as a straight anteroposterior film of the left upper quadrant should be obtained. There is no danger in giving barium orally in cases of small bowel obstruction, and one may find the etiology as well as the level of obstruction. A barium enema can be helpful in diagnosing large bowel obstruction (Figure 3–8), as well as in evaluating patients with massive lower gastrointestinal tract bleeding. Acute diverticulitis with perforation (Figure 3–12) and abscess formation can be diagnosed readily, as can perforation by a foreign body. In volvulus, a barium enema is often not necessary if the survey film is diagnostic. A barium enema is contraindicated if the survey film shows the characteristic distention of the transverse colon as-

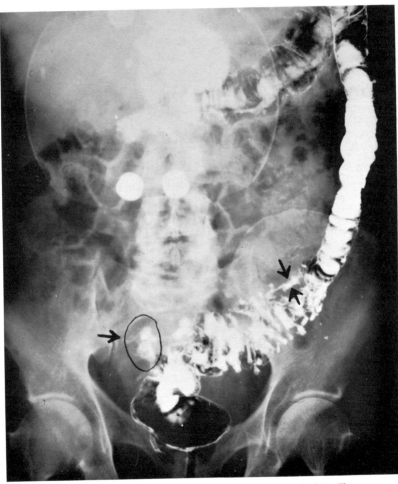

FIGURE 3–12 A barium enema study of diverticulitis. The arrow and circle indicate a perforation, and the two arrows point to an intramural abscess.

sociated with fulminating ulcerative colitis (toxic mega-colon). Intussusception can easily be revealed by barium enema. This examination has also been useful in the diagnosis of acute appendicitis in which the appendix does not fill and in which signs of pericecal inflammatory mass are often present.

An intravenous urogram is very helpful in evaluating patients with flank pain in whom ureteral calculus is suspected. Deviation of the right ureter can be seen in acute regional enteritis or appendicitis with abscess formation. Abnormal function, distortion of the collecting system, or delayed appearance of contrast medium on one side is very significant in patients with suspected renal trauma. A cystogram, in which a water-soluble contrast medium is injected into the bladder, is a valuable procedure in evaluating patients with pelvic fractures and hematuria to detect bladder or urethral injury.

The intravenous cholangiogram can be extremely useful in the evaluation of the acute abdomen. In the absence of previous cholecystectomy, the gallbladder should be visible by 1 or 2 hours after the examination has begun. Nonvisualization is presumptive evidence of obstruction of the cystic duct by stone or edema. Visualization of normal ducts and gallbladder all but rule out the biliary tract as the source of the patient's disease.

Radioactive scanning may, at times, be indicated in the diagnosis of the acute abdomen. This technique can be used to assess vascular injuries to the kidneys (Hg^{197}) or liver (Au^{198}). It may also be helpful in determining the etiology of intraabdominal masses; rose bengal I^{131} is cleared by the liver in 30 minutes and collects in the gallbladder. This fact may be used to determine whether a right upper quadrant mass is functioning

Text continued on page 51.

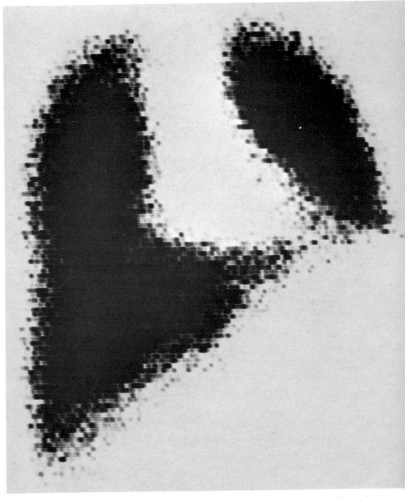

FIGURE 3–13 A normal lung-liver scan. Note that there is no free or clear area between the right lung and the liver.

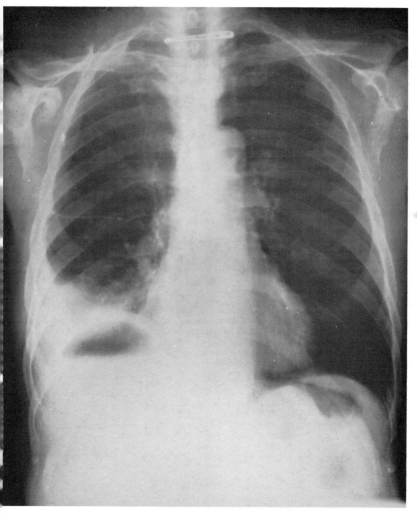

FIGURE 3–14 Upright film of the chest of a patient with a right subdiaphragmatic abscess and pleural effusion.

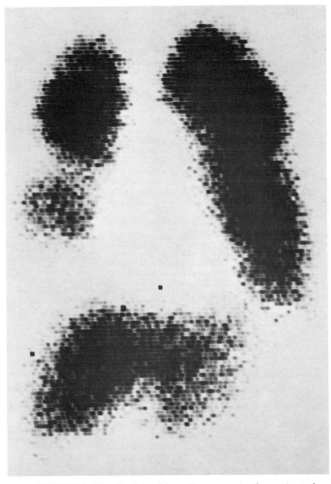

FIGURE 3–15 Combined lung-liver scan in the patient shown in Figure 3–14. Note the clear areas between the lung and liver as compared to those in Figure 3–13.

liver tissue or gallbladder. A liver scan (Au^{198}) may indicate the presence of liver abscess, cyst, or tumor and can be useful in the diagnosis of right subphrenic abscess (Figures 3–13, 3–14, 3–15).

The roentgenologic examination of the patient with an acute abdominal problem is incomplete without posteroanterior and lateral chest films. Right lower lobe pneumonia can mimic appendicitis, and free air under the diaphragm usually is best shown in the upright chest film. The state of the heart and lungs is of importance in pre- and postoperative management of the patient. Left renal pain often is associated with poor aeration and discoid atelectasis at the left lung base. Fluid in the left costophrenic angle may contain high amylase levels in cases of acute pancreatitis. The presence of mitral stenosis alerts one to the possibility of peripheral emboli. Chest fluoroscopy to check the diaphragmatic motion and to look for fluid in the pleural space is very helpful in evaluating a patient with a possible subphrenic abscess.

ULTRASOUND EXAMINATION OF THE ACUTE ABDOMEN

EDWARD H. SMITH, M.D.[*]

4

In the past few years, ultrasonography has become a widely used diagnostic tool in a variety of abdominal disorders. As a result of recent improvements in technology the examination can be performed rapidly, and being noninvasive does not involve the use of ionizing radiation. The organs of the abdomen can be visualized and readily identified, and information concerning their internal structure can be obtained. Moreover, unlike many radiologic procedures, ultrasonic evaluation is independent of organ function. These attributes make ultrasonic evaluation of the patient with an acute abdomen especially useful.

PRINCIPLES

Ultrasound consists of sound waves of frequency above 18,000 cycles per second, or above the range of the

---

[*]Associate Professor of Radiology, Harvard Medical School; Director, Onco-Radiology, Charles A. Dana Cancer Center, Boston.

human ear. In practice, frequencies of 1 to 5 million cycles per second (or MHz.) are employed. Brief electrical impulses are produced by a pulse generator, converted to pulsed ultrasound in the transducer, and directed into the object to be examined in the form of a narrow beam. When the beam strikes a boundary surface between tissues of different densities and sound velocities (acoustic impedance), such as between fat and muscle, a portion of the ultrasound beam is reflected as echoes. When detected by the transducer, these echoes are converted to weak electrical voltages that are then amplified and transmitted to a cathode ray tube, in which they are presented in the form of a corresponding series of dots. Since the velocity of sound in tissue is known, the distance from the boundary surface to the transducer can easily be determined. The portion of the beam not reflected continues until it strikes new reflective surfaces. In older instruments the dots presenting to the oscilloscope were stored on a special storage screen, coalescing to form a sectional image. Depending on the amplitude, the echo was either recorded or not recorded, with no variation according to its strength. Newer instrumentation allows grading of echoes according to amplitude, producing a "gray-scale" image. Cystic lesions are fluid-filled and contain no interface to reflect the sound beam; therefore they are free of internal echoes. Solid masses, however, demonstrate internal echoes and attenuate the beam far more than cysts, allowing differentiation in the great majority of instances.

The transducer is oriented and moved in the desired sectional plane so that ultrasonic sectional views are obtained. These sectional views are usually taken in at least two planes at right angles, most often longitudinal and transverse, but any angle is possible. The images formed on the monitor are recorded in a number of ways, most often by an attached Polaroid camera.

Dynamic imaging, obtained either by mechanical or electronic means, recently has become clinically available and appears quite promising. Actual moving images in "real time" are obtained, somewhat analogous to those provided in fluoroscopy, allowing rapid surveillance of the entire abdomen. Examination time is decreased and the examination is less dependent on the skill of the operator.

METHOD

The patient is placed on an examining couch, usually in the supine position, except when posteriorly accessible structures such as the kidney or tail of the pancreas are being imaged. Limited patient preparation is required. Since sound transmission through air (and bone) is minimal, large amounts of bowel gas may seriously interfere with the examination. By restricting intake by mouth and administering drugs such as simethicone, one occasionally can decrease the amount of intestinal gas and improve the quality of the examination.

Generous amounts of mineral oil are applied to the abdomen to insure optimal acoustic coupling. In general, longitudinal and transverse scans spaced 1 to 2 cm. are obtained, supplemented by other views when desired. An average examination takes approximately 30 to 45 minutes. It is important to stress that an ultrasound examination should precede a barium study, since residual barium interferes with sound transmission.

CLINICAL APPLICATIONS

GALLBLADDER AND BILIARY TREE

The normal gallbladder can be visualized when distended, so that the examination is performed after the patient has fasted. In acute cholecystitis stones, with rare exceptions, are present and can be identified in ultrasound diagnosis in a high percentage of cases (even when only a few millimeters in diameter) because of the great impedance mismatch between the bile fluid and the dense, compact stones. In addition to direct imaging of the reflected echoes from the surfaces of the stones,

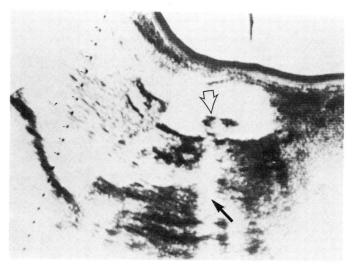

FIGURE 4–1 Longitudinal scan through gallbladder containing stones (*open arrow*) which appear as dense echogenic structures, strongly reflecting the sound beam, causing acoustical "shadowing" (*closed arrow*).

acoustical "shadowing" may aid in detection (Figure 4–1). Ultrasound can be utilized in cases in which oral cholecystogram is equivocal or not possible because of jaundice or poor liver function. In the latter circumstance, as high as 90 per cent of calculi can be identified.

In addition to the gallbladder, dilated intrahepatic biliary radicles may be identified, as well as a dilated common duct. The cause of extrahepatic biliary obstruction, such as a common duct stone or an extrinsic obstructing mass, may be discovered as well.

Certain conditions that mimic acute cholecystitis can be discovered by ultrasound examination. Accurate placement of a fine-gauge needle for transhepatic cholangiography can be accomplished under ultrasound

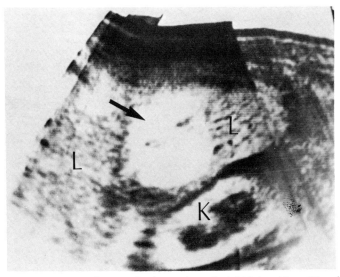

FIGURE 4–2 Longitudinal scan through right lobe of liver (L) and right kidney (K), showing echo-poor, rounded structure (*arrow*) due to abscess.

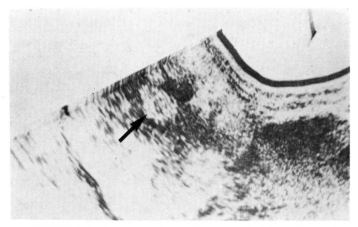

FIGURE 4–3 Longitudinal scan through right lobe of liver, with loss of normal homogeneous pattern and discrete structure (*arrow*) typical of metastases.

guidance using a specially constructed offset transducer with a central channel through which the needle is introduced.

LIVER

Occasionally a patient with a focal process in the liver may present with symptoms of an acute abdomen. A liver abscess (Figure 4–2; see description of abscesses further on) or large metastatic deposit (Figure 4–3) may be detected. Extrahepatic fluid collections such as ascites (Figure 4–4) or subdiaphragmatic abscesses (Figure 4–5) are also identifiable. Laceration, if the separation is large enough, may be seen along with extrahepatic hematoma formation. In cases of acute right-sided heart failure ac-

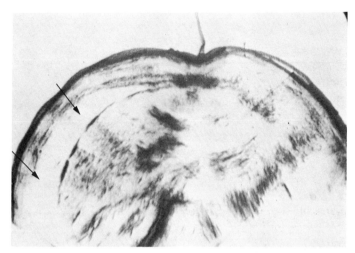

FIGURE 4–4 Transverse scan demonstrating echo-free fluid collection typical of ascites (*arrows*) surrounding lateral border of liver.

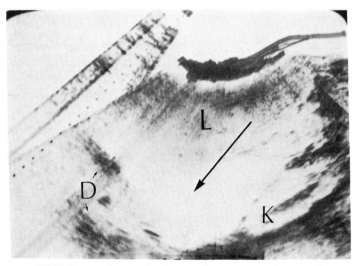

FIGURE 4–5 Longitudinal scan demonstrating large collection (*arrow*) under diaphragm (D) displacing liver (L) anteriorly and right kidney (K) inferiorly.

companied by severe right upper quadrant pain, hepatomegaly with dilated hepatic vein branches along with a dilated inferior vena cava may be an important clue to the underlying etiology.

PANCREAS

In acute pancreatitis, the entire pancreas may be enlarged and ultrasonically appear as a relatively echo-poor collar of tissue lying between the left lobe of the liver superiorly and the aorta, superior mesenteric artery, and inferior vena cava inferiorly (Figure 4–6). In many patients with acute pancreatitis physical examination of the abdomen is often difficult, and ultrasound examination may reveal the presence of a surprisingly large

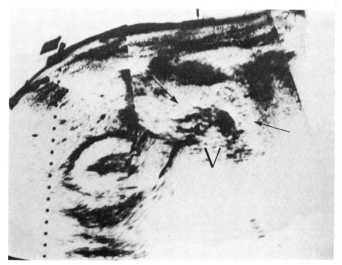

FIGURE 4–6 Transverse scan shows enlarged pancreas (*arrows*) straddling vertebral body (V).

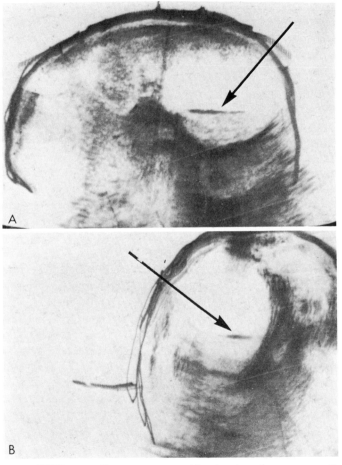

FIGURE 4–7 Transverse scan (*A*) showing large pancreatic pseudocyst with fluid-debris level (*arrows*) which is seen to shift on right lateral decubitus scan (*B*).

pancreatic pseudocyst which may not be palpable (Figure 4–7). If surgery is not undertaken, the progress of the lesion can be followed by sequential examinations to see if resolution occurs.

Occasionally, carcinoma of the pancreas may present with acute abdominal pain, and ultrasound may demonstrate a solid mass.

AORTA

The normal abdominal aorta may be readily visualized from just below the diaphragm to about the level of the umbilicus. Caudad to the umbilicus the bifurcation usually is obscured by intestinal gas.

In any patient presenting with a tender, pulsatile, midline mass, ultrasound examination should be performed immediately to identify the presence of an aortic aneurysm (Figure 4–8). Its size and extent and the presence of clot in the lumen can be precisely determined. If surgery is not indicated, sequential studies are performed in order to detect any increase in size.

Not infrequently, especially in elderly women with flaccid abdomens, a suspected palpable pulsatile mass is revealed by ultrasound examination to be a very superficially located, perfectly normal caliber aorta (Figure 4–8). In many institutions, aortography for aortic aneurysm is no longer routinely performed, the ultrasonic examination being considered the definitive study.

SPLEEN

The spleen can be well delineated by ultrasonography but the examination has to be individually tai-
Text continued on page 65

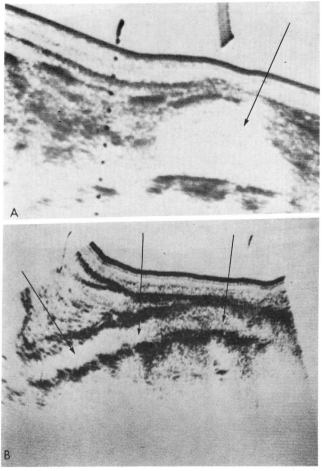

FIGURE 4–8 Longitudinal scan through abdominal aortic aneurysm *(A)* in contrast to normal but superficially located abdominal aorta *(B)*.

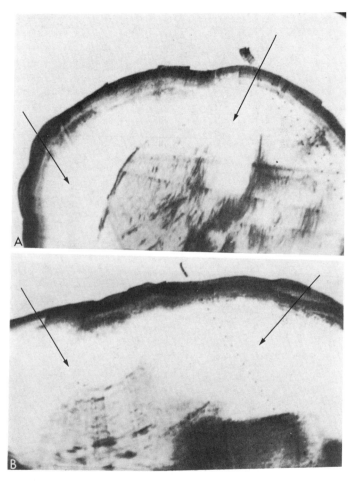

FIGURE 4–9 Transverse (*A*) and longitudinal (*B*) scans in patient
with massive intraperitoneal hemorrhage (*arrows*). The anechoic collection occupying most of the abdomen cannot be differentiated from
ascites or any other fluid collection.

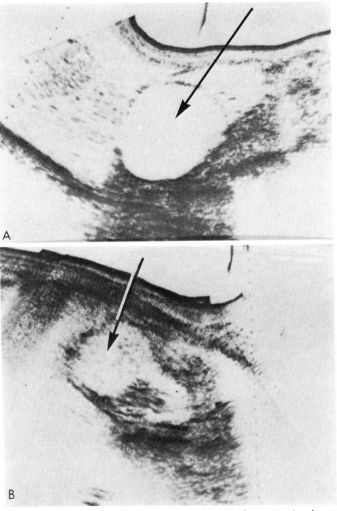

FIGURE 4–10 Longitudinal supine scan (*A*) demonstrating large, anechoic, sharply defined right upper pole renal cyst (*arrow*) adjacent to liver. This is in contrast to large upper pole echogenic mass (*arrow*) in left kidney in prone longitudinal scan (*B*) due to carcinoma.

lored in order to visualize the entire organ. Blunt abdominal trauma may lead to a subcapsular splenic hematoma, which may be identified ultrasonically, or to frank rupture with intraperitoneal hemorrhage (Figure 4–9). Subphrenic collections on the left may develop in a variety of clinical situations and may displace the spleen. Intrasplenic processes are rarely the cause of an acute abdomen but may present ultrasonically as a mass within the spleen.

KIDNEYS

Acute pyelonephritis or ureteral colic is not diagnosed by ultrasound but complications of these conditions may have characteristic ultrasonic appearances, as in perinephric abscess or hematoma. Calcifications within the kidney may be suspected on ultrasound examination but are diagnosed more readily by conventional radiologic studies. Occasionally an intrarenal mass may suddenly enlarge and present with acute symptoms, and differentiation between a cyst and a solid tumor easily may be made by ultrasound examination (Figure 4–10).

ADRENALS

The normal adrenals are usually too small to be identified by ultrasonography, but masses, whether primary or secondary, may be readily visualized if they are sufficiently large.

RETROPERITONEUM

Acute retroperitoneal collections or neoplasms can be readily delineated and their dimensions accurately mapped out. Retroperitoneal adenopathy, when over 2 to 3 cm. in size, can be identified by a typical ultrasound appearance, especially in the para-aortic area. Involved nodal areas not imaged by lymphography often can be visualized.

GASTROINTESTINAL TRACT

Common conditions affecting the gastrointestinal tract leading to acute abdominal symptoms, such as peptic ulcer with or without perforation or intestinal obstruction, do not lend themselves to ultrasonic detection, especially since they are frequently accompanied by large amounts of intestinal gas. In fact, a large quantity of free air from a perforated viscus may obscure the underlying structures, preventing an adequate ultrasonic study. Radiologic investigation should not be delayed in these situations. Complications of gastrointestinal disease such as appendiceal or diverticular abscesses can be detected by ultrasound examination.

ORGANS OF THE TRUE PELVIS

URINARY BLADDER.   In all examinations of the pelvis the patient should be instructed to arrive with a full bladder, which provides an ultrasonic "window" displacing the gas-filled small intestine. Acute urinary retention in

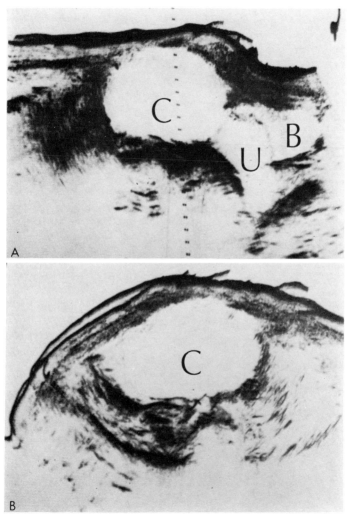

FIGURE 4–11 Longitudinal scan *(A)* through large ovarian cyst (C) superior to normal uterus (U) and bladder (B). Transverse scan *(B)* through cyst.

both males and females is an important condition to be kept in mind in a patient with acute abdominal distress. The overdistended bladder can be identified promptly on ultrasound examination and proper therapy can be quickly instituted.

OVARIES.   A distended urinary bladder must be distinguished ultrasonically from an ovarian cyst, which may twist or bleed and cause acute symptoms. When small, the lesion usually is located eccentrically, but when large an ovarian mass may occupy the entire pelvis and abdomen (Figure 4–11). A tubo-ovarian abscess also may be responsible for acute abdominal symptoms and may be diagnosed ultrasonically (Figure 4–12).

UTERUS.   Any patient of childbearing age with a pelvic mass and abdominal symptoms should have an ul-

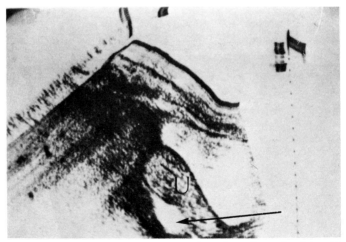

FIGURE 4–12 Longitudinal scan through midline of pelvis with anechoic collection due to an abscess (*arrow*) in the cul-de-sac, posterior to a normal uterus (U).

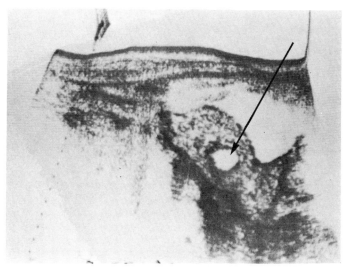

FIGURE 4–13 Longitudinal scan through the uterus demonstrating a gestational sac (*arrow*) age 6 to 8 weeks.

trasound examination prior to roentgen studies or initiation of potentially hazardous therapy in order to exclude the possibility of an intrauterine pregnancy. A gestational sac can be consistently identified after 6 to 8 weeks (Figure 4–13). Common conditions that present with similar clinical findings and often can be differentiated by ultrasound examination are ectopic pregnancy, tuboovarian abscess (Figure 4–12), and uterine leiomyoma.

INTRAABDOMINAL ABSCESSES

Abscesses may develop anywhere in the abdomen, may lead to acute abdominal symptoms, and may be very difficult to detect despite complex and often invasive examinations. Many patients have to undergo exploratory laparotomy as the ultimate diagnostic procedure. However, ultrasonic examination, often in conjunction with radionuclide scanning, is the method of choice in preoperative localization of occult abdominal abscesses.

In general, abscesses are typically echo-free or echopoor, but may have complex patterns due to fibrous septa or loculations. Because of their relative lack of internal echoes they are particularly suited for ultrasonic detection, especially when they are in typical (i.e., subphrenic or periappendiceal) locations and are of sufficient size (approximately 2 cm. in diameter) (Figure 4–5). However, since they may be present anywhere and are often multiple, careful examination of the entire abdomen in a systematic fashion often may be necessary. This is especially true in the postoperative patient, particularly when immunosuppressive therapy has been administered (e.g., after renal transplantation or chemotherapy for neoplasm).

ULTRASONICALLY GUIDED FINE NEEDLE ASPIRATION

As mentioned previously, under ultrasound guidance using a specially constructed transducer containing a central channel, a fine needle can be safely and precisely placed anywhere in the abdomen and a specimen obtained for cytologic and bacteriologic examination. In this way, a suspected diagnosis of malignancy, abscess, hematoma, or starch granuloma may be positively confirmed or excluded. The procedure is extremely safe and is preferable to blind needle insertion. In certain instances, a tissue diagnosis can be obtained and therapy instituted without resorting to exploratory laparotomy.

CONCLUSION

Ultrasonography has become an important tool in the diagnostic armamentarium and should be used in conjunction with other traditional methods, such as radiographic and radionuclide studies, to arrive rapidly at the correct diagnosis. The patient is subjected to the least discomfort and risk without compromising accuracy. The utility of ultrasound in the diagnosis of the acute abdomen has been reviewed and its limitations pointed out.

ARTERIOGRAPHY IN PATIENTS WITH THE ACUTE ABDOMEN

DAVID C. LEVIN, M.D.[*]

5

The use of arteriography as a major technique in diagnostic radiology dates back to 1953 when Seldinger, working in Sweden, developed the percutaneous method of catheter insertion into the abdominal aorta. With this development, arteriography became a much simpler procedure from a technical point of view and one that no longer required major surgery to accomplish. The current practice is to perform arteriography in patients who are lightly sedated. The principal site of arterial puncture is the femoral artery, although the axillary, carotid, brachial, and popliteal arteries and the aorta itself can be catheterized directly if necessary. An experienced arteriographer, equipped with the proper catheters and guide wires, can selectively catheterize most of the important arteries within the abdomen, frequently including second- and third-order branches.

*Co-director, Cardiovascular Radiology, Peter Bent Brigham Hospital, Boston; Assistant Professor of Radiology, Harvard Medical School.

In this chapter we will deal primarily with the application of arteriography to the evaluation of patients presenting with an acute abdomen. Gastrointestinal bleeding and traumatic injuries are the two acute situations that are most appropriate for arteriographic evaluation. Arteriography may also provide important information in the evaluation of other lesions such as ruptured abdominal aortic aneurysms, renal and splenic infarcts, intra-abdominal abscesses and hematomas, and ischemic bowel disease. Arteriographic aspects of each of these lesions will be discussed.

GASTROINTESTINAL BLEEDING

The principal role of arteriography in the patient with the acute abdomen is in the diagnosis and treatment of gastrointestinal (GI) bleeding, a technique pioneered in 1963 by Baum, Nusbaum, and their colleagues at the University of Pennsylvania. If bleeding originates from an artery, selective injection of contrast medium into the involved vessel will demonstrate extravasation into the gut. The extravasation is best seen during the late arterial or venous phases, and usually allows very precise localization of the actual bleeding site.

The ability of the radiologist to detect and localize GI bleeding is directly related to the rapidity with which it is occurring at the time of contrast injection. Early experimental studies suggested that bleeding at a rate of only 0.5 ml./min. was detectable. Further clinical experience has indicated, however, that in human patients a rate of 2 to 3 ml./min. is required for detection. Another important factor is successful manipulation of the catheter tip into a position as close as possible to the source of hemorrhage. Thus, for example, if a patient is bleeding from a duodenal ulcer supplied by a branch of the superior pancreaticoduodenal artery, a celiac axis arteriogram may fail to demonstrate it; however, if the catheter tip is advanced superselectively into the gastroduodenal artery (which gives rise to the superior pancreaticoduodenal), the bleeding site *will* be visualized.

The importance of proper clinical timing cannot be overemphasized. Arteriography should not be carried out immediately after the patient is admitted to the emergency room; frequently, the bleeding may have stopped spontaneously by that time or else will respond to initial medical therapy. After several hours of observation, it is usually possible to determine clinically whether the patient is continuing to bleed actively, and at that point arteriography should be considered. If a patient is bleeding actively when the procedure is performed, and if the angiographer can successfully position the catheter tip relatively near the source, accurate detection and localization of the bleeding should be possible in the vast majority of cases. A negative arteriogram usually is accompanied by clinical evidence of cessation of bleeding. In our experience at the Peter Bent Brigham Hospital, arteriography has detected the source of GI bleeding in 63 per cent of cases.

The most common sources of upper GI bleeding demonstrated by arteriography are Mallory-Weiss tears, erosive gastritis, and gastric or duodenal ulcers. The most common sources of lower GI bleeding at arteriography are vascular malformations (particularly in the cecum and ascending colon), colon diverticula, small bowel tumors, and Meckel's diverticula. Arteriograms shown in Figures 5–1 to 5–3 demonstrated the source of bleeding in three patients who were hospitalized for acute GI hemorrhage.

Text continued on page 80

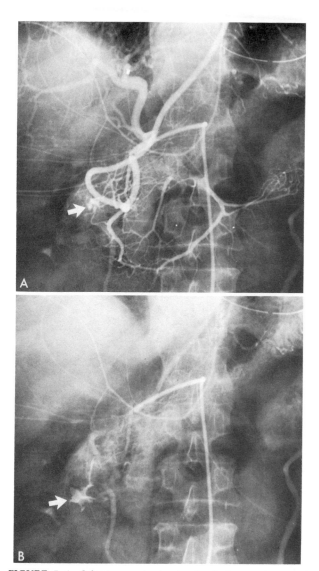

FIGURE 5–1 Selective gastroduodenal arteriogram in a patient with a bleeding duodenal ulcer. These early and late phase films show extravasation of contrast from a small arterial branch in the duodenum (*arrow*).

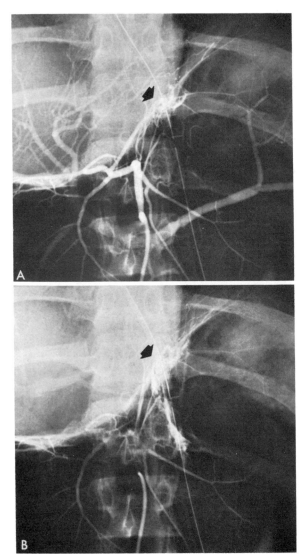

Figure 5–2 *Legend on the opposite page.*

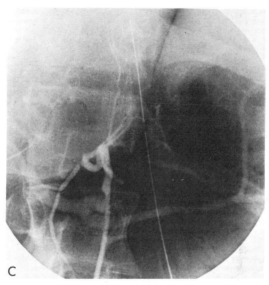

C

FIGURE 5–2   Arterial bleeding from the region of the gastroesophageal junction in a young man suffering multiple injuries from an automobile accident. *A* and *B*: Early and late arterial phase films from a selective left gastric arteriogram showing extensive extravasation of contrast (*arrowheads*) from a branch of the left gastric artery in the region of the gastroesophageal junction. *C*: Repeat selective left gastric arteriogram in the same patient following a 20-minute infusion through the catheter of vasopressin, 0.2 pressor units per minute. Note that the bleeding has stopped almost completely. Further infusion therapy resulted in complete cessation of bleeding. The bleeding did not recur, but the patient died 1 week later of peritonitis. Autopsy revealed a gastric rupture at this point.

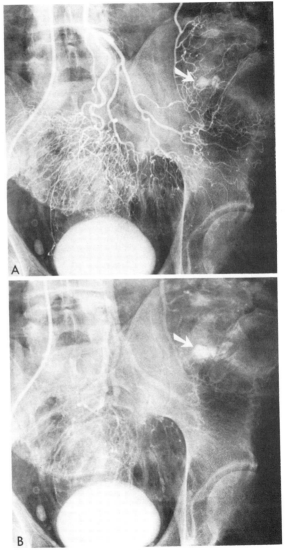

Figure 5–3 *Legend on the opposite page.*

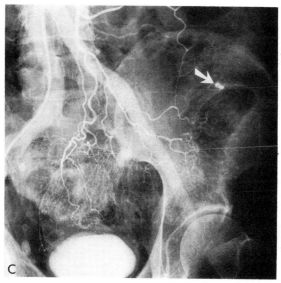

FIGURE 5-3 Massive lower gastrointestinal bleeding in an 80-year-old male. *A* and *B*: Early and late phase films from a selective inferior mesenteric arteriogram demonstrate considerable extravasation of contrast material (*arrows*) from a proximal sigmoid branch. *C*: Repeat inferior mesenteric arteriogram following a 30-minute infusion of vasopressin, 0.2 pressor units per minute. Note that the extravasation is considerably less pronounced, indicating response to the drug. The infusion was continued and the patient thereafter ceased to bleed altogether. No further bleeding occurred and the patient was eventually discharged without surgery.

Once the bleeding site has been localized, an attempt may be made to control it by infusion of vasoconstrictor drugs or injection of embolic material through the catheter. The most widely used vasoconstricting agent at the present time is vasopressin. This drug can be infused at a rate of approximately 0.2 pressor units per min. for a period of days. If necessary, a dose rate as high as 0.4 pressor units per min. can be used for shorter periods. Once there is clinical evidence that bleeding has stopped, the infusion should be tapered gradually; as a safety measure the catheter should be left in place for approximately 24 hours in case bleeding occurs again. Examples of successful treatment of GI bleeding by transcatheter vasopressin infusion are shown in Figures 5–2 and 5–3.

An alternative method of therapy is the introduction of embolic material (such as autologous clot or strips of Gelfoam) through the catheter to obstruct the bleeding artery. This method, if successful, has the advantages of stopping bleeding rapidly and does not immobilize the patient for hours or days, as occurs with placement of a catheter. The disadvantages are that it is irreversible and less controllable; the emboli may pass into vessels other than those which are bleeding. Transcatheter embolization is relatively safe when used for gastric or duodenal bleeding, since these organs have a rich collateral vascular supply which can prevent tissue necrosis. It is probably not safe for use in small bowel or colon bleeding, where collaterals are not as well developed, unless the catheter tip can be superselectively positioned directly in the branch supplying the site of extravasation.

Arteriography cannot demonstrate active bleeding from gastroesophageal varices, although the venous phase of celiac, splenic, or superior mesenteric arteriography usually shows the enlarged varicosities. If arterial hemorrhage is ruled out arteriographically in patients with known portal hypertension, varices can then be assumed to be the bleeding source. Vasopressin infusion into the superior mesenteric artery acts to constrict small bowel arteries, thereby decreasing inflow to the portal venous system, and helps to control variceal bleeding. Recent evidence has suggested, however, that intravenous vasopressin therapy may be just as effective in such patients.

In our experience at this hospital, in 61 per cent of all patients whose bleeding sites were arteriographically demonstrated, hemorrhage was controlled by transcatheter introduction of vasoconstricting drugs or embolic material.

TRAUMA

Arteriography has proved to be very useful in evaluating traumatic injuries of the solid abdominal viscera, especially the liver, spleen, and kidney. It is of somewhat more limited value in dealing with trauma of the pancreas or the intestine.

Blunt hepatic trauma may result in a variety of complex injuries with mortality of 30 to 70 per cent in reported surgical series. One of the principal reasons for this poor prognosis is that the surgeon often has difficulty defining the exact location, type, and extent of injury during the surgical procedure. Some of the more important types of hepatic injury are (1) subcapsular hematoma; (2) parenchymal rupture with hematoma formation; (3) contusion; (4) laceration or avulsion of blood vessels; (5) arteriovenous fistula; (6) pseudoaneurysm with hemobilia; and (7) traumatic bile cyst.

The subcapsular hematoma presents angiographi-

cally as an avascular mass that displaces the liver away
from the borders of the abdominal cavity and produces
an extrinsic compression deformity or concave outer
border at the liver margin. Parenchymal rupture with
hematoma formation also appears as an avascular mass,
but this time within the parenchyma. Hepatic arteries
and portal veins are stretched around the periphery of
the mass. Parenchymal contusion results in patchy hyper-
vascularity and irregular accumulation of contrast medium within liver tissue. Laceration of hepatic artery
branches causes extravasation of contrast medium during
angiography, similar to that which occurs in cases of gastrointestinal bleeding. Hepatic artery–portal vein fistulae
may develop within only a few hours following blunt
hepatic trauma. Angiography demonstrates direct flow of
contrast material from hepatic artery branches to portal
vein branches in such cases. A hepatic artery pseudoaneurysm appears as a saclike collection of contrast medium
which fills directly from an arterial branch. These lesions
result from laceration of an artery and subsequently may
decompress themselves by rupturing into a bile duct,
thereby producing hemobilia. A traumatic bile cyst results from interruption of a biliary duct and appears

FIGURE 5–4   Celiac arteriogram in a patient who had sustained
blunt hepatic trauma with intra-abdominal hemorrhage 1 month prior
to this study. The bleeding site was presumed to be a sigmoid diverticulum. He had continued to bleed despite two surgical attempts to control
it. These films demonstrate a pseudoaneurysm (*arrows*) arising from a
small branch of the left hepatic artery. This obviously represented the
source of bleeding. Just above and lateral to this lesion, there is a large
parenchymal rupture with hematoma formation and contusion. The
rupture and hematoma are manifested by stretching and lateral displacement of branches of the right hepatic artery and the large radiolucency
in this region seen on the late phase film. The patchy, mottled area just
under the right hemidiaphragm represents an area of contusion.

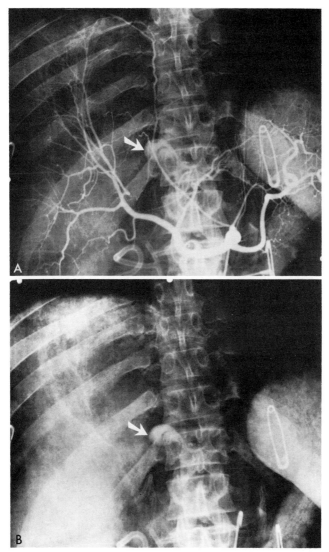

Figure 5–4 *Legend on the opposite page.*

angiographically as a rounded, sharply defined radiolucent area within the liver. Displacement of vessels around the border of the cyst may be present and the cyst wall may stain faintly with contrast medium during the late phase of the angiogram. These lesions tend to be more sharply circumscribed than parenchymal hematomas.

A patient was studied one month after blunt hepatic trauma (Figure 5–4) who had had two unsuccessful operations in the interval in an attempt to control bleeding from his liver. The angiogram demonstrated a large area of parenchymal rupture, contusion, hematoma formation, and the pseudoaneurysm that was undoubtedly the source of blood loss. Arteriography thus can define the nature and location of hepatic injury in many cases prior to the operation itself. It should be a part of the preoperative work-up in every patient who experiences hepatic trauma severe enough to suggest the need for surgical repair.

Splenic trauma is a much simpler problem from the surgeon's point of view. A seriously damaged spleen can be removed quickly without seriously affecting the future health of the patient. Obviously, this approach cannot be carried out in cases of liver injury. At angiography, a ruptured spleen may show extravasation of contrast material from arterial branches, pseudoaneurysm formation, or a defect in the parenchyma during the sinusoidal phase of the arteriogram corresponding to the area of parenchymal rupture. Figure 5–5 is an example of a patient who had a

FIGURE 5–5   Early and late phase films of a celiac arteriogram in a patient with a ruptured spleen. The lesion is best seen during the late phase and is manifested by a large irregular radiolucency (*arrow*) in the midportion of the splenic parenchyma. By contrast, note the normal, sharply defined margins of the upper and lower poles of the organ.

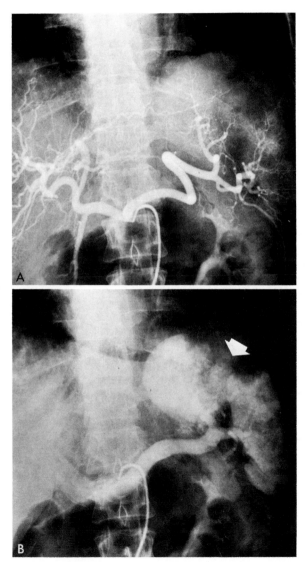

FIGURE 5–5 *Legend on the opposite page.*

parenchymal rupture of the spleen after falling on a stairway.

The arteriographic findings in renal trauma are similar to those in splenic trauma. Extravasation, psuedoaneurysm formation, and parenchymal rupture are all relatively common. Figure 5–6 is an example of a fracture of the kidney in a patient following an automobile accident. The intravenous pyelogram may be completely normal in some patients with renal parenchymal fracture.

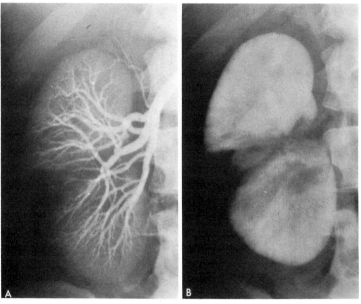

FIGURE 5–6 Early and late phase films of a selective right renal arteriogram in a patient with a fracture of the right kidney. Note the complete interruption of the parenchyma in the midportion of the kidney on the late phase film. In spite of this fracture, there was no angiographic evidence of arterial extravasation.

Pancreatic trauma may result in pseudoaneurysm formation, either directly as a result of damage to the artery or indirectly by leading to pancreatitis and subsequent digestion of pancreatic arterial walls as a result of the liberation of proteolytic enzymes. Arteriography can demonstrate both pseudoaneurysms and pseudocysts of the pancreas, although these studies rarely are required on an emergency basis unless active bleeding develops. Arteriography has not been used widely in the relatively rare circumstance of gut trauma, since most of these patients develop peritonitis rather than arterial injury. An unusual case of traumatic arterial injury of the stomach was demonstrated angiographically (Figure 5–2).

Treatment of traumatic lacerations of arteries and pseudoaneurysms by vasoconstrictor and embolic agents has been suggested and tried in some centers within the last several years. The results as yet are inconclusive, although definite benefits have accrued in some cases.

RUPTURED ABDOMINAL AORTIC ANEURYSMS

Rupture of an abdominal aortic aneurysm may be a rapidly fatal event if the rupture is large. Patients with aneurysms who develop small leaks, however, may present with an acute surgical abdomen. The diagnosis of an aneurysm often can be made noninvasively by a combination of clinical examination, plain x-rays of the abdomen, and ultrasonography. Arteriography confirms the diagnosis, but also supplies information that cannot be obtained by any other means. This includes the extent of the aneurysm, involvement of the origins of the renal arteries, and involvement of the iliac arteries. While this in-

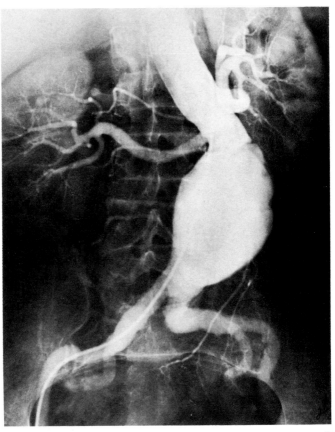

FIGURE 5–7 Large abdominal aortic aneurysm in a 67-year-old male. The aneurysm is well localized and does not involve either the renal arteries or the common iliac arteries.

formation is helpful to the surgeon, it may not be crucial. If the patient with a suspected ruptured aneurysm is in shock, or otherwise clinically unstable, he or she should be taken directly to the operating room without undergoing angiography. The angiogram almost never demonstrates the site of extravasation of blood from a leaking aneurysm, because of stasis of blood and laminated clot along the walls of the aneurysm. It is important to remember, therefore, that the absence of demonstrable extravasation of contrast material certainly does not rule out the possibility of a leak. An example of an arteriogram of a patient with a large abdominal aortic aneurysm is shown in Figure 5–7.

RENAL INFARCTION

Renal infarction is a common cause of an acute abdomen. If this diagnosis is suspected clinically, arteriography should be performed to confirm it. A main renal artery embolus usually can be demonstrated during an abdominal aortogram (Figure 5–8). The demonstration of smaller peripheral renal emboli requires selective catheterization of the involved renal artery. Renal emboli may originate from a variety of sources. These include thrombi in the left atrium in patients with mitral stenosis, thrombi in left ventricular aneurysms, vegetations on cardiac valves in patients with bacterial endocarditis, and thrombi on atherosclerotic plaques within the aorta. In a considerable number of patients with renal emboli, however, the source is not demonstrable.

The angiographic diagnosis of renal embolus can be

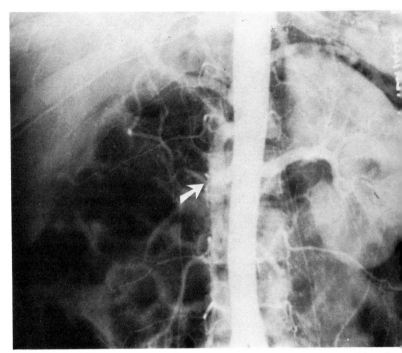

FIGURE 5–8 Right renal artery embolus in a 49-year-old female with mitral stenosis. The left renal artery and kidney are normal but there is an abrupt cutoff of contrast flow in the proximal portion of the right renal artery (*arrow*). No contrast material reaches the right kidney.

made if an abrupt cutoff of a major vessel is seen, in conjunction with lack of parenchymal opacification distal to the lesion. In cases of main renal artery obstruction, the lack of opacification will involve the entire kidney. If the embolus is segmental, the lack of parenchymal opacification will have a corresponding segmental configuration.

SPLENIC INFARCTION

Infarction of the spleen is considerably less common than renal infarction. These lesions have an angiographic appearance similar to that of renal infarcts, in that they are characterized by abrupt obstruction of a major or segmental splenic artery branch with a corresponding defect in opacification of the parenchyma.

ABSCESSES

Abscesses of various organs, such as the liver, kidney, spleen, pancreas, and adrenal, or of the retroperitoneal space, can present symptoms that closely mimic those of the more common acute abdominal crises. Fever is usually, but not necessarily, part of the clinical picture in these cases. Arteriography is performed only rarely in patients with acute abscesses but is employed frequently during the subacute or chronic phases. Intra-abdominal abscesses have a relatively consistent, but nonspecific, angiographic appearance, regardless of the organ of origin. A mass effect is usually seen, with displacement of vessels around its periphery. Fine neovascularity may be present, particularly at the border of the lesion. The demonstration of fine neovascularity may be somewhat confusing, since such vessels can be seen in both inflammatory and neoplastic masses. Coarse neovascularity is almost never seen with inflammatory masses and almost always signifies the presence of malignancy. In most intra-abdominal abscesses, even though fine neovascularity may be seen along the border of the mass, the main bulk of it remains avascular. In parenchymal organs that become well opacified during selective angiography such as the kidney, spleen, and liver, an abscess appears as a radiolucent filling defect during the late phase of the study.

HEMATOMAS

Bleeding from a nonatherosclerotic artery is an occasional cause of an acute abdomen. This complication sometimes occurs in patients on anticoagulant therapy, but in other cases the etiology of the hemorrhage remains obscure. Spontaneous hematomas may occur in the perinephric space, the retroperitoneal space, the pelvis, or between the leaves of the mesentery or omental ligaments. These hemorrhages are usually self-limited, caused by tamponade by surrounding soft tissues and organs. Arteriography rarely if ever demonstrates actual extravasation of blood from an artery, but does show displacement of nearby vessels by the mass of clotted blood. Although arterial displacement is a nonspecific finding, the correct diagnosis of a spontaneous hematoma should be suspected if it occurs in patients with unexplained blood loss outside the gastrointestinal tract.

ISCHEMIC BOWEL DISEASE

Acute mesenteric ischemia is characterized by severe abdominal pain, nausea, vomiting, diarrhea, distention, shock, and gastrointestinal bleeding, and is considered one of the most serious of acute abdominal crises. In earlier years, this disease was thought to be the direct result of arterial occlusion by thrombi or emboli. Less commonly, venous obstruction was postulated. More recently, the studies of Siegelman, Sprayregen, Boley, and their colleagues at Montefiore Hospital and of Wittenberg and Athanasoulis and their colleagues at the Massachusetts General Hospital have shown that a nonocclusive form of this disease also exists. About one-half of cases of small bowel ischemia are of the nonocclusive type, while over three-quarters of cases of colonic ischemia are nonocclusive. This discussion focuses primarily upon small bowel ischemic disease, since this is the more acute form; ischemic colitis tends to be a less virulent and somewhat more chronic clinical entity.

If small bowel ischemia is suspected clinically, arteriography can be performed in an attempt to differentiate the occlusive from the nonocclusive form. Emboli or thrombi that occlude the superior mesenteric artery or its branches can be demonstrated as filling defects or abrupt terminations of major branch vessels. Once the diagnosis of occlusive ischemia is established, embolectomy or reconstructive vascular surgery can be carried out in an attempt to restore normal blood flow. If this fails, the jeopardized bowel usually will have to be resected.

The nonocclusive form of small bowel ischemia is something of an enigma. This disease usually develops in a clinical setting of decreased cardiac output, such as occurs with congestive heart failure, shock, or cardiac arrhythmias. It also can occur with digitalis intoxication, since this drug is a potent mesenteric vasoconstrictor. A prolonged decrease in mesenteric blood flow presumably leads to reactive mesenteric vasoconstriction, which produces an even greater decrease in flow and sets up a vicious cycle. This vasoconstricted state may persist even after the primary cause of ischemia is relieved. Angiography will rule out the presence of occlusive lesions and demonstrate instead diffuse narrowing of the superior mesenteric artery, segmental constrictions that often are seen at the origins of jejunal and ileal branches, and narrowing and poor filling of small intramural branches. These findings are all angiographic manifestations of the vasoconstrictor reaction.

Nonocclusive mesenteric ischemia cannot be corrected by surgery, which should be utilized only as a last resort if actual bowel necrosis occurs. The disease is treated primarily by attempting to reverse the condition of low cardiac output or digitalis toxicity. A promising approach, which has been used so far only in a relatively small group of patients, is treatment of the disease by infusion of vasodilator drugs through a catheter selectively positioned in the superior mesenteric artery. An intra-arterial infusion of papaverine, 3 mg./min., is given for 20 min., followed by a single bolus injection of 30 mg. of papaverine. Repeat arteriography is then performed to see if the angiographic abnormalities have been reversed. If improvement is noted, the papaverine infusion can be continued at a rate of approximately 45 mg./hr. for up to 24 hr. Reversal of the ischemic symptoms has been documented in some cases using this regimen. The prognosis for patients with nonocclusive mesenteric ischemia is generally poor, and this appears to be a promising mode of therapy.

ANESTHESIA FOR THE ACUTE ABDOMEN

*LEROY D. VANDAM, M.D.**

6

Acute abdominal surgical disease in the large majority of cases implies that emergency operation will be necessary. The difference between this and an elective operation is that less time is available to prepare the patient for anesthesia and the procedure he or she must undergo. Time available ranges from immediate intervention in a catastrophe, such as the burst aortic aneurysm or hemorrhage owing to trauma, to problems that require time for establishment of a diagnosis—a question of appendicitis or possibly a complication of pregnancy. In any case, however, anesthetist and surgeon are working toward the same goal—that is, early and complete recovery of the patient from the illness. Each, therefore, must

*Professor of Anaesthesia, Harvard Medical School; Anesthesiologist-in-Chief, Peter Bent Brigham Hospital, Boston.

understand the other's problems, and there should be no standing on prerogative or ceremony. If it is not possible to wait and an operation is the most important element of resuscitation, anesthesia must be given despite incomplete restoration of the body's reserves. When delay is permissible, and this is always a considered judgment, every effort should be made to return body function to normal. This means that the chance for development of complications during operation and postoperatively will be diminished in keeping with the adequacy of treatment. Anesthesia and operation superimposed on an acute illness are life-threatening stresses that call into play a complex of adjustments requiring all the reserves that the body has to offer.

Patients about to undergo anesthesia are classified by anesthetists according to physical status, ranging from Class 1, in which there is no physiologic impairment, to Class 4, in which the derangements are severe and life-threatening, involving body systems essential for survival. A patient in Class 5 is moribund and given little chance to survive, but may require an operation on the off chance that there is something surgically correctable. The resulting surgical morbidity and mortality closely follow this classification. The extremes of age — the newborn infant or the octogenarian — add additional complicating factors. Note that the term physical status is employed rather than risk. Risk is always greater in an emergency, and physical status must be further defined by appending an E (for emergency) to the category. A classification such as this serves to alert the anesthetist to the gravity of the situation and permits the compilation of mortality data and comparison of statistics between one clinic and another. In this way each is speaking in terms of the same kind of patient. The reasons why the emergency operation adds to the risk are implicit in the remainder of this discussion. Since the surgical problems are presented in detail elsewhere, only anesthetic considerations are discussed here.

GENERAL PROCEDURE

As soon as an acute abdomen is suspected, the anesthetist should be notified — in all fairness to his or her role as a consultant. The contribution of the anesthetist to patient care preoperatively will vary according to the individual's training and experience, and the need for his or her advice is in inverse ratio to the wisdom and skill of the surgical team. But two heads are always better than one. It may be that the anesthetist only has time to rush to the operating room with patient and surgeons to perform the necessary resuscitative operation. Or the anesthetist may help with resuscitation in the emergency ward and accompany the patient through the necessary radiologic examinations on the way to the operating room. In any situation in which the patient's condition may deteriorate rapidly he should be moved to the vicinity of the operating suite where he can be closely watched while necessary treatment and diagnosis are carried out. The patient should not be moved unless it is fairly certain that he will not collapse on the way. This requires preliminary supportive treatment.

PREANESTHETIC CONSIDERATIONS

The anesthetist does better when mentally prepared, being able to assemble the necessary equipment and drugs and summon help for the complicated operation in which blood pumping, complex monitoring, and administration of a variety of drugs will be necessary. Most important is the need to see the patient, for the anxious patient wishes to know how he or she will be taken care of. Although patients seek little detailed information about the operation they may worry about how they will be put to sleep, whether they will awaken prematurely or at all, or whether they will experience pain or vomiting in the postoperative period. Assurance on these points goes a long way toward diminishing the amount of preanesthetic medication necessary to relieve the anxiety, and possibly lessens the depth of general anesthesia needed. Preanesthetic medication must be chosen in accordance with the anesthetic agent to be used, a matter of mature judgment, so that the patient will be given neither too much nor too little. Intramuscular injection is preferred in the acute situation, the standard drugs being a sedative and a belladonna derivative. Narcotic analgesics are required for pain or in conjunction with the projected use of nitrous oxide, thiopental, and a neuromuscular blocker. Dosage and choice of drugs are based on the patient's past experience with anesthesia, allergic history, and physical condition at the time. None may be needed in the elderly or comatose patient, a great deal in the husky alcoholic with pain.

During the interview and examination of the patient, the anesthetist can ascertain the following: problems with previous anesthetics; condition of the teeth; probability of a full stomach; and physical characteristics that may cause difficulty in giving the anesthetic, particularly those involving the airway. Every aspect of the history, physical examination, and laboratory examination is just as important to anesthetic management as it is to surgical care.

Permission for an operation performed on a minor must be granted by the nearest relative or guardian, while the adult is expected to grant his or her own informed consent. Minimal laboratory data should include a hematocrit determination, white blood cell count and differential, and urinalysis. Beyond the age of 40 or so, or if the history suggests a problem in the young patient, an electrocardiogram and x-ray of the chest are important to have. Other tests must be done in relation to need and time available: serum electrolytes, sodium, potassium, perhaps calcium; blood urea nitrogen; serum enzymes for diagnosis of pancreatitis; culture for bacteremia; liver function tests; arterial blood gases to detect pulmonary insufficiency; and pH for estimation of acid-base balance. In this clinic we have not felt that measurement of blood volume is useful, largely because of changing conditions in the acute situation, lack of satisfactory standards, and long experience with the problems encountered, and because practically all elements of the physical examination and laboratory work point to the degree of blood volume deficiency.

SPECIAL PREANESTHETIC PROBLEMS

Surgical illness is often superimposed upon a medical problem, particularly in the elderly in whom the acute abdomen is most life-threatening. Many surgical conditions are complications of a medical illness or require a differential diagnosis that might dictate medical rather than surgical treatment. Acute or recent myocardial infarction carries a high mortality. Congestive heart failure and cardiac arrhythmias must be gotten under control.

Some believe that there is a place for prophylactic administration of digitalis to prevent development of congestive heart failure or a rapid arrhythmia that could result in hypotension and coronary or cerebral insufficiency. Prophylactic digitalization is appropriate in the elderly patient with generalized arteriosclerosis or in the patient with an enlarged heart, a history or presence of arrhythmia, a past history of congestive heart failure, and possibly long-standing hypertension. In the emergency case, digitalization in the presence of fluid and electrolyte imbalance may be risky from the standpoint of toxicity. However, the prophylactic use of digitalis may be safer than intravenous use when a complication has already appeared. Furthermore, the positive inotropic action of digitalis is useful in counteracting the myocardial depressant action of general anesthetics.

The hyperglycemia of diabetes, especially with acidosis, requires vigorous treatment even if the operation is delayed more than is desired. The chronic alcoholic, though not intoxicated at the time, may convulse or develop delirium tremens postoperatively. Anticonvulsive medication preoperatively and administration of alcohol intravenously during the operation may prevent both complications. All this is to say that medical consultation and treatment are often essential and that time must be taken to achieve the best results.

Lastly, in the presence of abdominal trauma, its surgical treatment may require simultaneous treatment of a head injury or trauma to the chest and its contents.

COMMON PROBLEMS DURING INDUCTION OF ANESTHESIA

Although these problems are discussed individually, it will be apparent that all are interrelated.

THE FULL STOMACH

A full stomach poses the hazard of regurgitation and aspiration of food, drink, or gastrointestinal secretions. Aspiration of large food particles or large volumes of liquid causes asphyxia and rapid death. Lesser degrees of aspiration result in atelectasis and pulmonary insufficiency. Material of high acid content (pH less than 2.5) causes bronchospasm, inflammation, atelectasis, and pulmonary edema. Aspiration consequent to pyloric stenosis, with achlorhydria and bacterial proliferation, may be followed by lung abscess. Aspiration of blood is not uncommon in massive gastrointestinal bleeding. Thus, it is essential to prevent this complication. Aspiration already may have occurred in any patient with an acute abdomen who has diminished upper airway protective reflexes—the elderly, the severely depleted, or the semicomatose.

There is no safe rule whereby the stomach can be judged empty. Vomiting does not assure this; neither does a Miller-Abbott tube placed in the small intestine. A gastric tube draining well does not guarantee freedom from intestinal reflux. Intraabdominal disease and the associated anxiety interfere with intestinal propulsive movement both neurogenically and mechanically, so that food or drink taken many hours earlier may not have been digested. Narcotic analgesics depress smooth muscle activity, morphine particularly affecting peristalsis in the duodenum.

One cannot guarantee that the patient given local or regional anesthesia will not aspirate gastrointestinal contents, but certainly the tracheobronchial tree must be protected during general anesthesia. This is the reason for obligatory choice of endotracheal anesthesia in abdominal operations. In some cases it is possible to intubate the trachea under topical anesthesia. However, for the procedure to be successful, patient cooperation is required. A patient may not be emotionally up to this requirement; furthermore, he or she may cough, regurgitate, and aspirate during topical anesthetization. Thus, most anesthetists resort to rapid tracheal intubation following intravenous induction of anesthesia with an intravenous barbiturate and succinylcholine, a short-acting neuromuscular blocker. In the depleted state associated with the acute abdomen the major hazard is development of arterial hypotension, even with small doses of the barbiturate. Cardiac arrhythmias may result. Before proceeding, the patient's lungs are denitrogenated by breathing oxygen, and he or she is placed in a semisitting position to discourage regurgitation. Pressure is applied to the cricoid cartilage to occlude the esophagus. After the tracheal intubation, the endotracheal cuff is inflated to supply a tight seal and general inhalation anesthesia is begun.

DEHYDRATION AND DIMINUTION OF BLOOD VOLUME

Hypovolemia coupled with electrolyte deficiencies and acid-base disturbance is chiefly responsible for de-

velopment of hypotension during induction and maintenance of anesthesia. With vasoconstriction already
present, induction of general anesthesia results in decreased cardiac output, peripheral vasodilation, and consequent disproportion between the circulating blood
volume and the vascular space. In the elderly patient or
one with arteriosclerosis, even a brief episode of hypotension may cause coronary or cerebral ischemia.

Hypovolemia must be anticipated in every acute abdomen as a result of vomiting, diminished oral intake of
liquids, and further restriction of oral intake on entry to
the hospital. Gastric drainage and diarrhea are obvious
sources of fluid and electrolyte loss. Peritonitis with pro-
tein-rich exudate, hemorrhage, and fever with increase in
insensible water loss add to the deficit. Many findings in
the examination point to the extent of deficiency: dry
inelastic skin and tongue, rapid pulse and narrow pulse
pressure, arterial hypotension, elevated hematocrit,
oliguria and concentrated urine, elevated BUN, and the
distended abdomen with fluid and gas accumulation apparent on x-ray. Yardsticks for adequate replacement
with fluid and electrolytes are found in the improvement
of symptoms, signs, and laboratory values.

ELECTROLYTE AND ACID-BASE DISTURBANCE

The varieties and combinations of fluid loss that
occur in the acute abdomen account for the abnormal
serum levels of sodium and potassium and disturbed
acid-base balance found. Acidosis as indicated by diminution of arterial pH may result from a combination of
respiratory insufficiency with inability to eliminate car-

bon dioxide; diminution in renal excretory capacity; and the anaerobic metabolism associated with hypoxia, vasoconstriction, and fever. Disturbed serum potassium levels lead to cardiac arrhythmias, conduction defects, and alteration in neuromuscular transmission. Serum levels of potassium and sodium as well as acid-base values determine the extent of the myocardial and peripheral vascular response to endogenously released catecholamines as well as to sympathomimetic amines given. The overall result is a trend toward circulatory insufficiency superimposed on a diminished circulating blood volume. In addition to problems in maintaining blood pressure, the anesthetist experiences difficulty in reversing the effects of neuromuscular blocking drugs because of electrolyte deficiency. Postoperatively, hyponatremia may be evidenced by torpor, a general hypodynamic state and ileus.

PULMONARY INSUFFICIENCY

Today many patients approach an operation with a background of cigarette smoking, cough, chronic bronchitis, and obstructive lung disease. Such a history implies an increased risk of development of postoperative pulmonary complications — atelectasis and pneumonia. According to statistics, if one were to characterize the high-risk pulmonary patient, he would be an elderly male — a smoker with chronic bronchitis and emphysema undergoing operation for infection in the upper abdomen. The acute abdomen results in alveolar hypoventilation because of the high diaphragms associated with intestinal distention, splinting of the chest wall associated with pain, and accompanying grunting respirations. The work of respiration is increased by the extra respiratory effort, thereby adding to the demand for oxygen. Pulmonary embolization may have already occurred in the chronically ill. The lungs may be stiffened and compliance decreased in heart failure. All these problems produce acute pulmonary ventilatory insufficiency. The resulting hypoxia and hypercarbia add to circulatory instability because of the greater demands on the circulation and adversely affect the response of the heart and peripheral vessels to endogenous catecholamines.

The possibility of further progression of pulmonary insufficiency postoperatively is a strong argument for tracheal intubation and carefully monitored ventilation intraoperatively carried into the postoperative period. If time permits, the patient should be introduced to intermittent positive pressure ventilation before the operation since this may be necessary postoperatively. As one cannot rely upon cyanosis as an indication of hypoxia and the signs of hypercarbia are elusive, repeated analysis of arterial blood for oxygen and carbon dioxide provides the best index of ventilatory sufficiency.

ALTERATIONS IN BODY TEMPERATURE

Elevation of body temperature may be the result of dehydration, peripheral vasoconstriction and lack of sweating that diminish heat loss; warm and humid climates add to the heat retention. However, the usual cause of hyperpyrexia is infection. Fever increases body metabolism, thereby placing further demands upon the circulation and respiration. It is well known that hyperpyrexia may cause convulsions, a not uncommon complication when general anesthesia is given to the dehydrated, acidotic child. For these reasons if time can be spared, body temperature should be lowered by means of surface cooling, hydration, and use of appropriate drugs. During the operation a cooling blanket and ice bags strategically placed will help to keep the temperature down. Use of anesthetic techniques that decrease body metabolism and induce heat loss is necessary: regional anesthesia such as epidural or spinal, open or semiopen breathing systems that permit heat loss, and the use of curare and anesthetics such as halothane that decrease overall body metabolism.

HYPOTHERMIA. Paradoxically, when modern anesthetic techniques are used in air-cooled operating rooms a more common result is accidental body cooling, with temperatures in some instances recorded as low as 92 or 93° F. Postoperatively it is not unusual, following a prolonged operation, to observe shivering and rectal temperatures in the range of 96 to 97° F. in a patient undergoing otherwise uncomplicated elective surgery. This comes about as a result of use of the anesthetic techniques just mentioned and exposure of the body and open body cavities to the cool environment. Accidental lowering of the body temperature, unlike deliberate hypothermia, does not prevent the normal response to cooling, which consists of shivering and peripheral vasoconstriction. Such a response may elevate body metabolism as much as 200 or 300 per cent, adding considerably to the demands upon the circulation and respiration. Therefore, an attempt should be made to maintain body temperature at a normal level by avoidance of unnecessary exposure, the use of warming blankets, and warming bank blood of changing temperatures.

APPROACH TO ANESTHESIA

ESSENTIAL DRUGS

In view of the many physiologic derangements that may result from an acute abdomen, the following pharmaceuticals and drugs should be available before anesthesia is begun.

1. Replacement fluids, each with a purpose: dextrose in water; lactated Ringer's solution; saline; a variety of electrolyte solutions; and whole blood or its components.

2. Vasopressor drugs. Bearing in mind the disadvantages to their use, these drugs are used in the emergency to maintain the blood pressure until the basic problem is corrected. The aim is to maintain cerebral and myocardial perfusion in the vulnerable, the aged, and those with vascular disease. Depending upon the nature of the circulatory abnormality, a drug is chosen for its pharmacologic effect. A sympathomimetic amine may exert positive inotropic and chronotropic actions on the heart, or peripherally, to produce vasoconstriction at the arteriolar level and capacitance vessels, or a combination of both actions. The pressor may be given as a single intravenous or intramuscular injection or by continuous infusion. A good selection of drugs should include: metaraminol (Aramine) with central and peripheral actions; mephentermine (Wyamine) with central effects and possibly lesser peripheral vasoconstriction; phenylephrine (Neo-Synephrine) with largely peripheral actions; and, when the pressure cannot be elevated by treatment directed toward the cause, levarterenol (Levophed) or isoproterenol (Isuprel).

3. Hydrocortisone either for suspected adrenal insuf-

ficiency or for the pharmacologic effect in treating refractory types of hypotension that accompany endotoxin shock.

4. Drugs for heart failure and cardiac arrhythmias: digoxin; lidocaine; and procainamide.

5. Mannitol to induce diuresis and prevent development of acute tubular necrosis.

6. Bicarbonate to correct metabolic acidosis and for resuscitation from cardiac arrest.

7. Antibiotics at the surgeon's request.

MONITORING

In connection with the abnormalities listed, the following are procedures and techniques useful in the care of the critically ill; their use usually is extended into the postoperative period.

1. Auscultatory measurement of blood pressure or auscultatory monitoring of heart sounds with a thoracic or esophageal stethoscope.

2. Several intravenously placed catheters for administration of anesthetics, supportive drugs, and replacement fluids, inserted percutaneously or by cutdown.

3. Monitoring of the electrocardiogram on an oscilloscope and provision for recording of the electrocardiogram should accurate diagnosis be necessary.

4. Measurement of central venous pressure via catheter inserted percutaneously or by a surgical cutdown, the location confirmed by electrocardiographic tracing, pressure measurement, or fluoroscopy. The purpose is to measure venous pressure as influenced by circulating blood volume, fluid replacement, venous distensibility,

overall capacity of the circulation, and the performance of the heart. The central venous line is also used for administration of fluids and drugs, but care must be taken because a drug given via this route reaches the central circulation in higher concentrations than via peripheral routes.

5. An intraarterial catheter percutaneously or surgically placed for continuous monitoring of systolic, diastolic, or mean arterial blood pressures as well as for sampling of arterial blood for blood gas and acid-base analysis.

6. Thermocouples or thermistors placed in the nasopharynx, esophagus, or rectum for recording body temperature.

7. Catheterization of the urinary bladder for observation of urinary output and measurement of specific gravity.

8. Other equipment should include a mechanical ventilator, for the anesthetist finds it difficult to carry on artificial ventilation of the lungs simultaneously with the many other things he or she must do. The adequacy of ventilation and the function of the ventilator are monitored by observation of movement of the chest wall and analysis of arterial blood for oxygen, carbon dioxide, and pH.

Measurement of the hematocrit provides insight into the oxygen-carrying capacity of the blood when electrolyte solutions rather than blood are used in replacement.

ANESTHETIC MANAGEMENT

Recovery from anesthesia depends largely upon the preparation of the patient and intraoperative and postoperative management, as noted. There is no one anesthetic agent or technique that is best for any particular problem. Each anesthetist should choose that which he or she does best. Essentially what is needed is a quiet relaxed belly so that the surgeon can do the work easily and rapidly. Poor operating conditions add to the risk.

REGIONAL VERSUS GENERAL ANESTHESIA

LOCAL ANESTHESIA

Carefully given local anesthesia by infiltration, field block, or intercostal nerve block may be the safest method of all, but comparatively few procedures can be done this way with comfort for the patient. In local anesthesia, problems with toxicity of the local anesthetic arise as well as reactions to the epinephrine used. Comparatively short surgical procedures can be done satisfactorily with infiltration or field block: gastrostomy, cecostomy, enterostomy, transverse colostomy, or peritoneal drainage.

SPINAL OR EPIDURAL ANESTHESIA

Spinal anesthesia provides excellent operating conditions because of the quiet abdomen, the contracted bowel, and the relaxation that results from interference with sensory and motor transmission in spinal nerves. The amount of local anesthetic required is small and of no pharmacologic consequence. Disadvantages include: an awake patient; the high level of anesthesia required to block afferent visceral sensation; the inability to avoid retching and vomiting in operations done high in the abdomen; the resulting high sympathetic block that usually causes profound hypotension in the presence of hypovolemia; the poor alveolar ventilation if the lower intercostal nerves are paralyzed and retractors are used beneath the diaphragms; the unprotected airway; the serial injection of the local anesthetic required for prolonged operations; and the hyperperistalsis caused by sympathetic blockade that may lead to leakage at the time of an intestinal anastomosis, fecal discharge through an enterostomy, or defecation on the table. Epidural anesthesia offers the same operating conditions as spinal anesthesia.

GENERAL ANESTHESIA

General anesthesia calls for protection of the airway and controlled ventilation of the lungs. Although minimal general anesthesia is often sufficient in the depleted patient, the requisite degree of abdominal muscle relaxation in other patients can only be reached with deep anesthesia and at the price of severe circulatory depression. In most cases a combination of light general anesthesia with a neuromuscular blocking drug is used. As the patient improves during the operation, as he or she will when hemorrhage is controlled and fluid losses are replaced, the requirement for anesthetic increases, an encouraging sign.

POSTOPERATIVE CARE

Although a patient may have emerged safely from anesthesia and been set upon the course to recovery by the operation, the postoperative period is crucial and more demanding from the standpoint of time and stress imposed. The central nervous system, respiration, circulation, liver, kidneys, and endocrine glands are put to the test. Thus, the same considerations noted for the preoperative and intraoperative phases apply to postoperative care. Intensive postoperative care of the critically ill patient is merely an extension of the observation and treatment carried out during anesthesia and operation.

PITFALLS TO AVOID IN DIAGNOSIS OF THE ACUTE ABDOMEN

7

The chief pitfall in the diagnosis of the acute abdomen is the tendency to depend primarily on therapeutic weapons and to rely less on accurate diagnosis. Diagnostic acumen must keep pace with therapeutic power if the patient is to benefit. The practitioner must have pride and confidence in his or her ability to interpret the patient's problem. At the same time the physician must be humble enough to realize that there are pitfalls to avoid in the diagnosis of the acute abdomen.

Many mistakes made in the diagnosis of the acute abdomen are due to typical human error. The majority of these mistakes are of three types. First, the error of neglecting to take an adequate history and to perform a physical examination. This error is indefensible. Second, the error of commission; the patient is examined, but significant abnormal findings are disregarded or missed. This mistake is comprehendible but certainly undesirable.

Third is the error of erroneous interpretation of abnormal findings. This is much more subtle. It is the pitfall that even the most experienced must guard against. These are the basic pitfalls, and in the following discussion we apply them to the examination of the patient who presents with acute abdominal disease.

THE HISTORY

When the patient describes his pain he may be poorly equipped in vocabulary or at a loss for words because the pain is a new and unique experience. The doctor must put words into the patient's mouth, and in so doing must employ words of the right kind. Often the patient is asked if the pain is steady, or if it "comes and goes." However, a few patients with abdominal pain feel that it never really "goes away" and say that it is there all the time. But if the doctor asks if it is "colicky or crampy," the patient may be able to equate it with a familiar experience, perhaps from childhood, and may answer in the affirmative, steering the physician toward the diagnosis of obstruction of the gastrointestinal, genitourinary, or biliary tract.

"Where is the pain?" is often asked; but where it was when the episode started, and where it is now give more helpful information. The pattern of midabdominal pain moving to the right lower quadrant in appendicitis is well known, but epigastric pain moving to the groin and testis in ureteral obstruction is often missed, along with the prognostic sign that the stone is moving. Abdominal pain moving to the back is thought of in pancreatitis, but often forgotten in pancreatic tumor or dissecting aneurysm. Right upper quadrant pain with referral to the shoulder calls cholecystitis to mind, but must also evoke the question of perforated ulcer, myocardial infarction, pneumonia, or pneumothorax.

"How long has the pain been there?" usually draws an answer of hours to days, and the doctor is satisfied. But further questioning will discover the nagging sensation in the pelvis, present for months, caused by an ovarian cyst that is now twisted and has become an acute problem. The obstructing sigmoid carcinoma presenting acutely as an obstruction with crampy pain may often have a history of months of tenesmus and rectal discomfort. Acute right lower quadrant pain in a patient with suspected appendicitis may be accompanied by a history of weight loss and diarrhea because of a right colon carcinoma that has now perforated. Thorough questioning may unearth a chronic problem that has finally presented as an acute abdomen.

"How is the pain affecting you?" should tell the physician something of the organs involved. A patient with abdominal pain who is hungry probably has disease elsewhere than the gastrointestinal tract. A few questions about eating, bowel movements, micturition, and menstruation do much toward localizing the diagnosis. The pitfalls of history taking are those of omission. The few examples given show how the well-phrased question and orderly sequence help to avoid them.

THE PHYSICAL EXAMINATION

Too often the physical examination of the acute abdomen amounts only to "feeling the belly," and the diagnosis is missed. Nowhere do the time-proved practices of observation, auscultation, percussion, and palpation pay greater dividends.

First observe the patient, then his or her abdomen. The patient who lies quietly, motionless, and barely breathing is avoiding the pain of an irritated peritoneum. The patient who is rolling about trying to find a comfortable position usually has pain caused by a distended viscus. The pitfall of incomplete observation misses much information and often the whole diagnosis. The abdomen must be completely exposed. An incarcerated femoral hernia may be missed if the groin is covered by a bedsheet or roll of fat. The splinted chest wall, the bruised flank, and the rash of herpes zoster may be covered by a cotton sheet over the patient or a sheet of ignorance in the physician's mind. Observation in a darkened room is a pitfall of the neophyte, who will miss jaundice, abdominal splinting, chest splinting, and visible peristalsis.

Auscultation of the heart has received so much attention that refinements in murmurs can be purchased on records and learned like a language. Conversely, auscultation of the abdomen is practiced and understood by very few. One of the obvious reasons is that the abdomen does not give out 72 sounds a minute and so one must listen longer. The "silent abdomen" may well be quiet for the 5 seconds that the observer allows, but if he listens longer the occasional peristaltic tinkle may indicate tube decompression and avoid a hasty operation.

The great pitfall in percussion is that it is not often done. Yet it tells in a moment whether the distended abdomen is filled with gas or ascitic fluid. It tells the examiner if the urinary bladder is distended. It shows if the liver dullness is obliterated by free air in the peritoneal cavity. Light percussion can be the gentlest way to identify localized abdominal tenderness.

Palpation requires a learned hand, but more often the truth is that palpation requires a warm, gentle, and patient hand. The cold hand finds spasm where there is none. The rough hand finds tenderness where there is no tenderness, and the patient hand finds the mass where the hurried hand finds only spasm. Incomplete palpation is fraught with danger. The groin is felt, but the inguinal ring is not palpated and the hernia is missed. The rectal examination is inconvenient, so the patient with a fecal impaction is sent to the hospital with a false diagnosis of intestinal obstruction. The pelvic examination is skipped and valuable information is missed.

Thus one can see that the pitfalls in physical examination are largely those of omission and incompleteness. Often one more question, another moment with the stethoscope, or obtaining adequate light and exposure will help the physician to avoid these errors.

PRIOR MEDICATION

The unrecognized effect of prior medication on the patient with acute abdominal disease who faces a possible surgical operation is a pitfall that every physician can avoid.

1. Adrenal steroid hormones are widely administered for many conditions, including inflammatory disease of the large and small intestine. Adrenocortical atrophy occurs after prolonged use of these drugs, and acute

adrenal insufficiency may develop when the patient undergoes the stress of a surgical operation. These patients can be operated upon safely, provided that extra intravenous adrenal steroid hormones are given during the operation and postoperative period. The other important effect of adrenocorticosteroids is that signs of acute inflammation may be masked; pain, pulse rate, leukocytosis, and temperature elevation may be diminished and unreliable in the presence of a serious intraabdominal inflammatory disease. The patient should be questioned specifically as to his or her intake of adrenal steroid hormones during the previous year to avoid this error.

2. Broad-spectrum antibiotics are frequently and often indiscriminately prescribed. They may mask the usual reaction to acute inflammatory abdominal disease and make the physical signs dubious. A careful history should be taken of what antibiotics the patient has taken recently and for how long.

3. Analgesic medications of varying strengths may have been taken by the patient prior to being examined for an acute abdominal condition and may modify his or her reaction to pain. It is helpful to the examiner if the type and amount of medication are known. Abdominal pain that is relieved by an aspirin tablet is probably not severe, whereas if morphine or a comparable drug has been given, the physical signs of a serious condition may be lessened. This pitfall is probably not as serious as formerly thought, since analgesic drugs do not change the course of the disease. They may delay diagnostic decisions, however, since the temporary pain relief must be allowed to wear off. If the analgesic has antipyretic action the patient's temperature may also be an unreliable sign of an existing inflammatory condition.

LABORATORY STUDIES

The laboratory examination is a complement to history taking and physical examination. It will give answers, but it won't ask the questions and hence is studded with pitfalls. The high hematocrit may be indicative of plasma loss in intestinal obstruction or mesenteric vascular accident, but a glance at the old record may show it is merely due to polycythemia vera or chronic pulmonary disease. The low hematocrit does not usually reflect acute bleeding but more often chronic disease. The normal hematocrit lures many into a false sense of security. A patient in hypovolemic shock may have a normal hematocrit simply because not enough time has elapsed for hemodilution to have occurred. The white blood cell count, too, may lead to many errors. A differential count may erase the security that the normal total count gives. A shift to the left is a basic sign of acute infection. Repeated white blood cell counts over a period of 6 to 12 hours may be the guiding sign in questionable abdominal conditions.

"We couldn't get a urine sample" is a pitfall that leads to mistaken diagnosis in renal disease. Red blood cells in the urinary sediment should suggest consideration of intravenous urograms to delineate injury, obstruction, or infection. If the patient is not able to pass a urine specimen and is acutely ill, the bladder should be catheterized both for urinalysis and to record urinary output.

"The abdominal film was unremarkable" is a pitfall that many stumble into. Was an upright film taken to show air-fluid levels not apparent on a flat film? Were the diaphragms included in the upright film to show air trapped beneath them? Conversely, was the entire pelvis shown to demonstrate a stone in the lower ureter? Was a chest film taken of the patient with upper abdominal pain to rule out pneumonia? Only when physician, radiologist, and technician work together can these pitfalls be avoided.

ABDOMINAL TRAUMA

SECTION 2

THE INITIAL APPROACH
TO THE PATIENT

8

Traumatic injury taxes the acumen of the most experienced surgeon. Injuries are frequently multiple, the patient may be unconscious, and many associated life-endangering problems may exist. Any type of lesion to any organ in any degree of severity may have occurred. The surgeon must consider all possibilities when diagnosing and treating abdominal wounds.

The major decision on the part of the surgeon examining the injured patient is whether or not operative intervention is indicated. This decision will probably be predicated upon making a specific diagnosis as to which organ or what part of the abdomen is injured, but the final decision must be whether or not an exploratory operation is required even if the exact site of injury cannot be ascertained. The placement of the incision will, in part, depend upon the site of injury, but even this can be rather non-specific, since a paramedian incision permits extension in either direction for exposure of the entire abdomen and its contents.

When caring for the patient who has sustained a traumatic injury, one must anticipate the worst rather than underestimate the extent of injury. When a patient is first seen after trauma to the abdomen, careful attention should be paid to his or her vital functions and signs before any specific examination is carred out so that the surgeon will be prepared to face any rapidly deteriorating situation that might arise.

If abdominal trauma is a part of a generalized injury, then other important considerations in the resuscitation of the patient should be dealt with before considering the abdomen. Primary attention must be given to the airway. Its patency is essential; if necessary, mouth-to-mouth breathing, insertion of an endotracheal tube, or a tracheostomy must be carried out to preserve adequate airway for survival. Cardiac function must also be evaluated rapidly and appropriate steps taken for any cardiac resuscitation that may be required. Along with cardiac function, there must be stabilization and replacement of blood volume deficit and careful attention to the vital signs (blood pressure, pulse, and respiration). One or more cutdowns for the administration of blood and other fluid should be placed immediately. A catheter for central venous determinations is of great value when there has been a large blood loss because it permits the surgeon to transfuse sufficient blood for volume replacement. The best clinical criteria for restoration of circulating volume in addition to the central venous pressure are the patient's pulse, blood pressure, and urine output. Stability of the chest and relief of any tension pneumothorax, hemopneumothorax, or sucking chest wounds all take priority over abdominal problems except for possible gross evisceration or major external abdominal arterial bleeding. Once the patient's general condition has been evaluated and stabilized, then and only then can the surgeon become involved with the diagnosis of abdominal injury.

The history of the accident and the mechanism of the actual trauma may be helpful in identifying the specific site of injury as well as in determining what action the surgeon should take. There are essentially four types of abdominal injuries.

BLUNT TRAUMA

This type of trauma is produced by a nonpenetrating injury such as that caused by a steering wheel, a moving object, a blow received in a fist fight, or a blunt instrument such as a stick or similar object. As demonstrated in Figure 8–1, this may be the most insidious type of abdominal injury. There may be absolutely no visible signs of injury exteriorly or at best a mild abdominal skin bruise or ecchymosis. If the patient is unconscious, there may be no appreciation whatsoever that the abdomen has been traumatized. Blunt trauma is the most common type of abdominal injury that presents to the surgeon and physician. The history of a blow, the knowledge of the direction of the blow, any bruising or ecchymosis, or localized complaint on the part of the patient must be heeded with great care. Even the most minimal physical signs may render abdominal exploration mandatory in patients who have suffered blunt abdominal trauma.

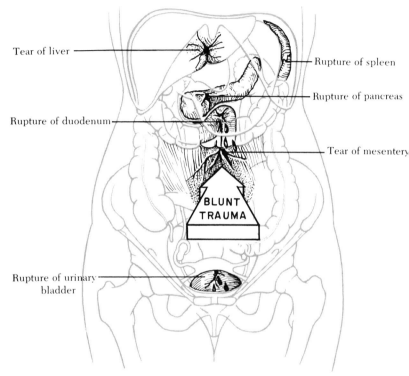

Tear of liver

Rupture of spleen

Rupture of pancreas

Rupture of duodenum

Tear of mesentery

BLUNT
TRAUMA

Rupture of urinary
bladder

FIGURE 8–1 Examples of specific injuries from blunt trauma.

STAB WOUNDS

Stab wounds are caused by a sharp instrument, usually a knife, ice pick, or a piece of metal or glass in an accidental injury. There is always a wound of entry, usually not a wound of exit. The wound of entry will give a key to the organs or tissues damaged (Figure 8–2). If possible, the direction of entry should also be ascertained. Stab wounds in the upper abdomen, in which the instrument of injury has been pointed in a cephalad direction, may enter the chest and produce cardiac injury despite a seemingly innocent epigastric wound.

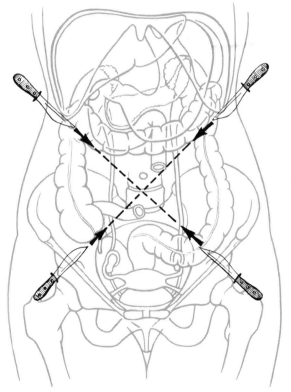

FIGURE 8–2 Stab wounds of the abdomen may cause injury anywhere in the peritoneal cavity and also in the chest.

Stab wounds must be explored without hesitation. There is no accurate way for the examining surgeon to ascertain the depth of the wound, and it is of little value to probe the wound with this in mind. As soon as the patient can be prepared for surgery, with his vital signs stabilized, he should have an exploratory laparotomy at which whatever organs or tissues are damaged should be appropriately repaired. It is better not to explore through the incision of the injury but rather to use a clean incision.

Wound sinograms are occasionally of help but they are painful and make subsequent examination of the abdomen difficult. They can also be misleading and falsely reassuring. The sinogram is performed by inserting a small Foley catheter into the wound and injecting radiopaque material into the tract of the wound. There must be a watertight seal at the point of entry of the catheter through the skin. A sinogram should not be done in multiple stab wounds and is unnecessary in instances in which intraperitoneal injury is clinically obvious.

GUNSHOT OR MISSILE WOUNDS

The gunshot wound may be very diffuse, especially if obtained in war, and large areas of the abdominal wall may be destroyed and gaping. There are also often associated blast and shock wave injuries (Figure 8–3). These, like stab wounds, must always be explored. There are often wounds of exit as well as entry related to gunshot or missile injury. Foreign bodies must be searched for; these may consist of the missile itself or clothing and other substances which may have been on the surface of the patient's abdomen before the missile

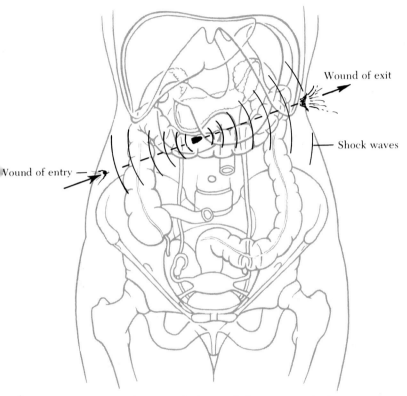

FIGURE 8–3 Gunshot wounds frequently have a wound of exit and also set up shock waves.

drove them forward into the abdominal cavity. The danger of other injuries such as to the chest or the spine from a single missile must be thoroughly considered, and the tract of entry and exit will indicate the areas that must be carefully examined. There is the additional danger of transmitted energy producing an expanding lesion upon contact with the abdominal surface or the surface of entry, which must be taken into account in treating any missile wound.

SHOCK WAVE CONCUSSION INJURY

This is the least common of the four types of injury, but it may be present with any of the other three, usually with gunshot or missile wounds. The pure shock wave concussion injury, of which a flash explosion is a good example, is one in which there is a blast wave but no actual contact with the patient by any missile. This makes the diagnosis extremely difficult, and reliance must be placed on the pertinent history and physical findings that tend to indicate perforation of a hollow viscus. In addition to primary viscus injury, there may be vast mesenteric injury with such a shock wave. As with blunt injury, close observation and a high index of suspicion on the part of the surgeon are necessary in the proper management of these patients. The force that such a shock wave, even from a great distance, can exert is phenomenal and should never be underestimated. The most commonly ruptured organs are the stomach, large intestine, and bladder, especially if any of these is distended, since the shock wave will be transmitted to the contents of any distended viscus.

GENERAL POINTS IN THE PHYSICAL EXAMINATION

1. The abdomen, perineum, and back should be examined thoroughly for any wounds or lacerations. These

can conceivably be either wounds of entry or exit. With any missile wound a most careful search must be made for a wound of exit or else the missile must be identified remaining within the body.

2. Any bruising, skin discoloration, or identifying marks that could give evidence of an abdominal injury should be searched for on every patient who has a history of trauma or who is unconscious.

3. Deformities of the rib cage, pelvic bone, and spine should be searched for as a key to any intraabdominal injury that might be associated.

4. Any abdominal distention or asymmetry of the abdomen may be the clue to intraabdominal injury.

5. Abdominal spasm, either voluntary or involuntary, with associated muscular rigidity may be the first sign noted on physical examination of a patient with trauma to indicate intraabdominal injury. This is particularly true in blunt trauma or shock wave injury in which so many other injuries may have occurred.

6. The presence or absence of bowel sounds to auscultation is an important part of the abdominal examination, especially as a baseline for future examination. In a patient with abdominal trauma who is under observation, the disappearance of bowel sounds that may have been present initially can be an ominous sign.

7. The finding of a mass is always significant and in the face of trauma usually indicates bleeding or an abdominal fluid collection. Enlargement of any of the organs or loss of their normal outlines, such as the percussible edge of the liver, may be of equal importance.

8. The digital rectal examination will aid in evaluating injury to the urethra, prostate, urinary bladder, and gross pelvic deformities from the trauma.

9. In any bleeding, the volume lost should be carefully estimated. The abdominal wall itself can bleed profusely; if bleeding can be controlled by a pressure bandage, an immediate differential can be made to determine whether it is coming from the abdominal wall or from within the abdominal cavity. These types of injury may, of course, coexist. Any drainage or seepage from a wound will provide important information about the site of intraabdominal injury. The presence of bile, gastric juice, intestinal contents, stool, or urine must always be sought in any abdominal wound.

RADIOLOGIC AIDS IN THE DIAGNOSIS OF ABDOMINAL TRAUMA

The role of radiologic examination of the acute abdomen is discussed in Chapters Three, Four, and Five. Radiologic examination of the severely injured patient may have to be withheld until the patient's condition is stable enough to tolerate being moved to the x-ray department unless x-ray films can be made with portable equipment.

LABORATORY AIDS IN INJURIES TO THE ABDOMEN

Certain laboratory tests greatly aid in evaluating and managing injured patients. One of the most important is the hematocrit. It may not be accurate when there is acute blood loss that is being replaced by transfusions. With a chronic blood loss the hematocrit falls as hemodilution occurs; this may be noted in the patient observed over many hours for signs of intraabdominal injury.

The hematocrit is most useful in the diagnosis of acute plasma loss. This takes place when there is major peritoneal injury, particularly rupture of the intestine, strangulation of the intestine, or traumatic pancreatitis in which there is an acute transudation of plasma into either the peritoneal cavity or the intestinal loops. The plasma deficit may be calculated accurately from the comparison of the normal and observed hematocrits and the patient's normal blood volume (Chapter Two).

Both the white blood count and the differential count are helpful in the patient being observed over a period of hours or days for the possibility of abdominal injury, but, of course, are of little value in the initial acute situation. Analysis of the urine is most important when the question of renal, ureteral, bladder, or urethral injury is present. Any patient with major trauma should have a catheter inserted when first seen. Not only is the quality of the urine important, but also the quantity of urine produced is a guide to the general status of the patient and his or her response to injury.

Lactic dehydrogenase (LDH) and other measurable enzymes in the serum, particularly the serum amylase, may be indicative of tissue injury. The amylase level indicates pancreatic damage, whereas the LDH and SGOT (serum glutamic oxaloacetic transaminase) may indicate bowel or liver injury. However, the correlation of the LDH elevation with specific injury to the intestine or other organs is still lacking.

In the acute abdomen of trauma, the use of the four quadrant abdominal tap may also be very useful when other criteria do not definitely indicate a diagnosis of visceral injury requiring exploration. This is particularly true in blunt and shock wave concussion trauma.

PREPARATION OF THE PATIENT FOR EXPLORATORY SURGERY

Just as the physician first seeing a patient after trauma must always suspect the worst, so the operating surgeon about to explore the abdomen of a patient with trauma or suspected trauma must always be prepared for all eventualities. One or two intravenous lines should always be in place. Adequate blood and plasma should be matched and available for immediate use. As much baseline information as is feasible should be obtained, including electrocardiogram, chest x-ray, serum electrolytes, blood urea nitrogen, blood sugar, and serum amylase and other enzymes. The operative procedure must not be delayed, but careful planning can often permit an adequate workup without being particularly time consuming. If the patient has had multiple transfusions before coming to surgery, evaluation of his or her bleeding and clotting factors, and the utilization of intravenous calcium and fresh blood should be considered. Blood volume determinations and central venous pressure measurements can be useful when practical.

It is most important that the patient's circulating volume be restored adequately prior to the operation because the addition of anesthesia to trauma may precipitate the rapid deterioration of the patient's homeostatic responses if replacement has been inadequate. Careful measurement of the urinary output as well as the central venous pressure, in addition to blood pressure, pulse, and respiration, may provide the key in the clinical setting to the degree of volume replacement. The use of mannitol often may be indicated intraoperatively if large blood losses are anticipated. Antibiotic as well as antitetanus therapy should be considered as a preoperative adjunct. The time and effort taken to resuscitate the patient and restore his or her homeostatic mechanisms as completely as possible prior to anesthesia and a surgical procedure are fully justified. The patient's instability will, therefore, not limit the management of whatever injuries are encountered on the operating table, and definitive therapy will be possible. Finally, consultation with others of the same discipline and other specialties should be freely utilized as needed.

SPECIFIC INJURIES FROM ABDOMINAL TRAUMA

9

LIVER

The liver is the abdominal organ most commonly injured, not unexpectedly, since it is the largest organ within the abdomen. Injuries of the liver can vary from small sharp lacerations to jagged stellate wounds, necrotic lobes, or massively fragmented lobes that bleed profusely. Massive hemorrhage occasionally occurs from a laceration caused by a percutaneous needle biopsy of the liver. The danger from liver injuries lies in uncontrolled blood loss or in the bile loss that will occur and will continue to occur long after the bleeding has stopped. Since the liver lies against the diaphragm, any wound of the liver must be construed as a potential wound of the chest cavity or the pericardial cavity as well, and the wound of exit from the liver should be sought, particularly in any stabbing injury. Any upper abdominal tenderness, spasm, or evidence of intraabdominal bleeding can be considered as coming from the liver and demands immediate exploration to control the site of bleeding. Small hepatic wounds can be controlled with large plication sutures and drainage. For massive hepatic damage, a formal lobectomy, right or left, is most appropriate. Recently hepatic artery ligation has been advocated as a simple and effective method of managing massive hepatic injuries.

An important late complication of hepatic injury is abscess formation. A foreign body driven into the liver substance can serve as a nidus for abscess formation, as can necrotic hepatic tissue inadequately debrided in a large laceration. Supra- or infrahepatic collections of blood or blood and bile also serve as the perfect focus for subphrenic abscesses.

SPLEEN

Because the spleen is such a friable organ it is often damaged in any type of abdominal trauma. Once damaged it bleeds profusely and must be removed. It is essentially impossible to control bleeding from the spleen with any assurance in any other way. Although the spleen may be damaged, the bleeding into the free peritoneal cavity may be delayed for a period of days or weeks because the bleeding may extend beneath the capsule (subcapsular rupture). Then at a later time, as the hematoma enlarges, it will rupture into the free peritoneal cavity and produce symptoms. The initial episode may produce left upper quadrant abdominal pain that may subside, and many of the signs may disappear only to recur at a later date when least expected.

The findings include fractured ribs on the left, unexplained acute blood loss with hypovolemia or shock, pain in the shoulder as evidence of diaphragmatic irritation on the left, left upper quadrant spasm, and absence of peristalsis (Figure 9–1). X-ray examination may be very helpful. The abdominal tap, particularly in the left upper quadrant, may be useful.

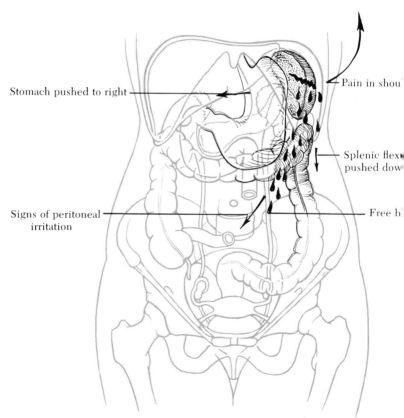

Stomach pushed to right

Pain in shou

Splenic flex
pushed dow

Signs of peritoneal
irritation

Free b

FIGURE 9–1   The symptoms and signs of a ruptured spleen.

Associated injuries to the stomach, pancreas, or left kidney may occur with splenic injury and should always be searched for at the time of operation. An important consideration in the operative management of the ruptured spleen is the rapid elevation of the spleen from its fossa so that the vascular pedicle can be controlled. Although this may be lifesaving, the surrounding organs must be protected. A paramedian incision is generally used rather than a subcostal incision, since it gives more rapid access to the abdomen and greater freedom to approach other organs that may have been damaged.

STOMACH

It is unusual for the stomach to be damaged by blunt trauma since it is thick-walled, very mobile, and generally high in the abdomen. This, however, may not be true if it is distended from a recent meal. Rupture of the stomach usually causes marked upper abdominal rigidity, possibly localized to one side or the other. Often free air is present, peristalsis is absent, and severe pain is present if the patient is conscious. The stomach frequently is injured by gunshot or stab wounds because it is fixed at the esophageal and duodenal end and cannot slither out of the way as the small intestine often will do. The blood supply to the stomach is so rich that it is rarely necessary to resect much gastric tissue; rather, it is possible just to debride the edges of the wound and to close it primarily, usually around a gastrostomy tube. If there is a high gastric lesion in which there is a possibility that the vagus nerve fibers may have been injured, it is important to perform a drainage procedure in the pyloric area after the wound is repaired. It is entirely possible to do this as a second stage.

PANCREAS

Injury of the pancreas is common with blunt trauma, since it overlies the spine and is an immobile organ. It can also be damaged, along with the spleen, in its more lateral portion, or even may be damaged during splenectomy for a ruptured spleen in which it may be difficult to identify the tail of the pancreas. The usual sequela to a traumatized pancreas is either pseudocyst associated with traumatic pancreatitis and rupture of ducts to the surface of the gland or a pancreatic fistula. Pseudocysts may be self-limiting and initially may be observed to see if they will subside; if continued pain, continued elevation of the serum amylase, and progression of the size of any upper abdominal mass thought to be a pseudocyst occur, then surgical management will be necessary (Figure 9–2). The age of the pseudocyst in part determines surgical management. A fairly fresh cyst with a thin wall may be treated by external drainage in the hope that the ductal connection will fibrose and the cyst will "dry up." The long-standing pseudocyst from trauma is best treated by internal drainage either to the stomach, if it is in close approximation to this organ, or to a loop of jejunum by a Roux-en-Y type of anastomosis. In general, marsupialization to the outside is a dangerous procedure because it provides an opportunity for the patient to rapidly develop metabolic acidosis as a result of the selective loss of bicarbonate in the highly alkaline pancreatic juice.

Pancreatic fistulas must be treated by adequate drainage, preferably with a sump drain, since it is almost

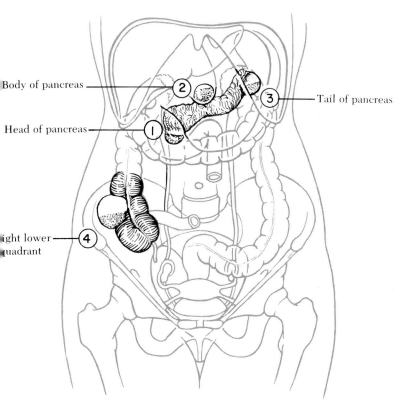

Body of pancreas

Head of pancreas

Tail of pancreas

ight lower
quadrant

FIGURE 9–2   The frequency (1, most frequent...4, least frequent) and location of pancreatic pseudocysts.

impossible to find the specific site of injury in the pancreas. It is important that the tract be kept open until the pancreatic injury does heal or until internal drainage can be established. If the skin portion of the fistula closes too early, abscess or pseudocyst formation is certain to occur.

The role of limited, immediate resection of damaged portions of the pancreas is being reconsidered.

Traumatic pancreatitis usually is associated with deep pain radiating through to the back, but on exploration may often be difficult to diagnose. There may be extensive bleeding into the retroperitoneum, rapid development of retroperitoneal edema, and many other associated intraabdominal injuries. It may not be until the postoperative period, when leakage of pancreatic juice is detected from the wound, particularly one that has been drained, that the diagnosis of pancreatic fistula can be made. The ability of the juice to digest the emulsion from x-ray film or a piece of catgut suture may often make the diagnosis. Multiple pseudocysts and multiple areas of trauma to the pancreas may be present simultaneously, and so much peripancreatic reaction may develop that portal vein hypertension may actually be noted on an acute basis in patients with traumatic pancreatitis. On some occasions the abdominal tap may produce fluid that has a very high amylase concentration, which again indicates traumatic rupture of pancreatic ducts into the free peritoneal cavity.

Any patient in whom pancreatic injury is suspected should immediately be placed on nasogastric suction, should be given antibiotics, and should be observed carefully for any evidence of plasma volume deficit. Plasma and albumin are important in the early management of this volume deficit, which can cause shock.

KIDNEY

Although mobile and surrounded by a cushion of fat, the kidneys are vulnerable to blunt trauma, particularly in contact sports and automobile accidents. Lying in the retroperitoneal space as they do, a great deal of perirenal bleeding can occur before detection by physical examination. Distention or discoloration of the flank may often be the first evidence of renal injury. The urine should be carefully examined for gross and microscopic bleeding in any injury, but on occasion bleeding may be so severe that renal shutdown may occur or clots may block the renal pelvis or ureter so that no blood comes into the bladder from the injured kidney. Clots in the ureter may produce renal colic indistinguishable from that of ureteral stone, and this may help provide the diagnosis. Unexplained ileus may also be present in renal injury. The mechanism and path of the injury may give an important clue to whether or not it is likely that the kidney has been damaged. Rupture of the kidney may tear the parietal peritoneum overlying it and, therefore, cause profuse intraabdominal bleeding. Ultrasound scanning and angiography may be very helpful in the diagnosis (Chapters Four and Five). The kidney should always be carefully palpated and examined in any intraabdominal exploration for trauma.

In addition to leakage of blood from a ruptured kidney into the free peritoneal cavity, urine also may leak into the peritoneal cavity or the retroperitoneum, especially in trauma in a patient with a hydronephrotic kidney in which there is a distended renal pelvis. This can produce gross peritonitis with all its physical signs. Trauma to one kidney can produce acute tubular necrosis in that kidney, and aortography may be necessary to establish whether the renal vasculature is patent. The danger of bilateral acute tubular necrosis from a unilateral lesion is always a possibility, especially when such diagnostic procedures as intravenous pyelogram, retrograde pyelograms, and aortography are added to the injury.

At the time of operation every attempt should be made to preserve renal tissue. If the kidney is so hopelessly fragmented that any preservation of renal tissue would leave a poorly vascularized kidney and would offer opportunity for hypertension, nephrectomy should be performed. Nephrectomy must never be carried out until it has been ascertained that a normal functioning kidney is present on the other side and that the injured kidney is not solitary.

Ureters rarely are injured by blunt trauma but may be damaged by gunshot wound or other missile injury. They also may be damaged during abdominal exploration of a generalized injury because identification in a damaged retroperitoneum may be a serious problem. Unrecognized damage to the ureters may lead to anuria, which is one of the indications for cystoscopy and retrograde pyelography in such posttraumatic cases. If ureteral injury has occurred in the course of trauma, unless there is very little loss of vascularity and continuity of the ureter so that direct repair is possible, a nephrostomy, as the initial treatment, should be undertaken followed by later plastic repair of the ureter. The most important consideration about ureteral injury is to recognize it.

SMALL INTESTINE

The small intestine is vulnerable to all four types of trauma mechanisms and may be damaged in multiple sites; therefore, in any exploration of the abdomen for trauma the entire small intestine must be examined carefully on all its surfaces before the surgeon is satisfied that it has not been damaged. Small intestine injury, aside from the presence of any intestinal contents on abdominal tap or free air on abdominal films, may be detected by the loss of liver dullness owing to air overlying the liver, the presence of diffuse abdominal rigidity, loss of peristalsis, rebound pain, and the general findings of diffuse peritonitis. Intestinal injury may not declare itself immediately. That is, the small bowel may be damaged by blunt trauma, and the wall may become infarcted and the bowel subsequently perforate. Whenever possible, because of its good blood supply, small bowel injuries may be debrided and closed primarily with or without enterostomy. Fistula formation may occur after small bowel injury if the exact extent of devitilized bowels is not recognized and the damage repaired at the time of exploration.

LARGE BOWEL

Trauma to the colon is common because the attachment of the large intestine in both the right and left gutters leaves only the transverse colon and the sigmoid freely movable. Since the large intestine often is filled with gas, the concussive type of injury may cause spontaneous rupture. However, the usual injury is from a stab or missile wound. These injuries may be lethal because of the widespread peritonitis that rapidly develops. Fecal drainage may often be detected either coming through the wound directly or upon abdominal tap, and the signs of severe peritonitis appear rapidly. Another type of trauma, especially in war, is that of the perineal wound in which the wound of entry enters the abdominal cavity through the perineum, passing through the rectum or sigmoid. Self-inflicted trauma to the rectosigmoid is always possible in disturbed persons; sigmoidoscopy or anoscopy often aids in this diagnosis.

Whereas with small intestine injury it is frequently possible either to close the wound directly or to carry out a short primary resection, large intestinal wounds require a quite different type of surgical management. The available techniques for the surgical management of the injured colon are by necessity varied, and one must choose the safest method to fit the particular site and extent of injury. In general it is good surgical judgment to make a proximal diverting colostomy regardless of the type of repair made distally. The options the surgeon has to choose from are as follows: (1) primary closure of a small wound in the colon can be done but should not be attempted in the presence of massive tissue damage or gross fecal peritonitis, (2) primary repair of the defect plus a proximal colostomy, (3) exteriorization of the loop of injured bowel, (4) resection and primary anastomosis are more applicable to injuries of the right colon, (5) resection and primary anastomosis with a proximal colostomy or enterostomy, and (6) resection with end colostomy and either a distal mucous fistula or Hartmann closure of the distal end. This last procedure is useful in injuries of the left and sigmoid colon. If the wound is fairly clean it may be debrided and closed, but a defunctionalizing colostomy always should be placed proximal to any wound of the colon. If the wound is badly contaminated the damaged bowel itself can be exteriorized. Perineal wounds involving the rectum can be drained widely through the posterior approach. Treatment of right-sided colonic wounds generally consists of emergency colectomy, proximal decompression with enterostomy and a direct ileotransverse colostomy. In addition, the area around any wound must be widely drained even if it is closed primarily and appears to be clean. One other difficult problem in the management of trauma to the large bowel is evaluating the viability of the tissue over a short interval of time. The small intestine, with its far superior blood supply and increased metabolic requirements, declares its state of vascular insufficiency within minutes. With multiple injuries involving the mesentery of the large intestine and perivascular hemorrhage, often an accompaniment of injury to the bowel itself, the dangers of any primary closure, even with apparently adequate debridement, are magnified. It is often possible to ascertain the degree of viability by the actual bleeding from the cut surface of the bowel, and in large bowel injuries this may be the best practical key to viability.

OMENTUM AND MESENTERY

The omentum is rarely damaged because it is so mobile. It can, however, bleed profusely if one of its vessels is lacerated. Although it is freely movable, it may be the first structure to be fixed and immobilized by adhesive bands. Damage to the omentum necessitates its resection. However, the omentum is always valuable both for plication of wounds of the intestine, spleen, liver, and pancreas, and often to protect the wound closure itself.

Damage to the mesentery can be insidious and it may accompany any of the types of abdominal trauma. When the abdomen is explored for injury, not only should the bowel itself be carefully examined, but its mesentery as well. Large hematomas may develop and progress in the base of the mesentery and eventually produce thrombosis and secondary infarction of bowel that previously has looked perfectly viable. Attempts to control bleeding mesenteric vessels that have retracted into the fat may produce further damage to bowel as more of the arcades require ligature. This is especially true in older persons in whom collateral circulating channels already may have been called into play during the natural history of their vascular disease. Another important concept in managing mesenteric injuries of a traumatic nature is the need to reexplore the abdomen if any evidence of progressive bleeding becomes apparent. It may be impossible to identify all bleeding points at the time of the initial procedure, particularly when hypovolemia is present. Although hemostasis may have been adequate, as the blood pressure is restored secondary hemorrhage from the torn mesenteric vessel that had been in spasm or inadequately perfused may occur over a matter of hours after the injury. Continued blood loss and contracting circulating volume as evidenced by poor urine output, decreased blood pressure, and rising pulse rate are warning signs for the surgeon to reenter the abdomen. This is one of the most commonly unidentified types of trauma when multiple other injuries are present, such as ruptured spleen, liver, or obviously ruptured intestine.

BLADDER

Injuries to the bladder are common in many types of trauma. Automobile accidents frequently cause pelvic fractures, and the splintered pelvic bones may easily puncture the bladder and then return to normal bony configuration without much displacement by the time an x-ray is made. If there is any evidence of blood in the urine, poor urine output, or peritonitis that is otherwise unexplained, a cystogram should be taken as soon as possible through a transurethral catheter. In the male, it is essential to precede this with a rectal examination to be sure that the prostate is in the normal position. Both prostatic rupture or displacement and rupture of the bladder can occur with pelvic fracture. Extravasation of tremendous quantities of urine into the retroperitoneum can occur with a great deal of hemorrhage and may be missed for hours or days if it is not thought of. Shock wave and blunt trauma may also produce rupture of the bladder, particularly if it is distended at the time of the injury. Peritoneal tap sometimes may reveal urine within the peritoneal cavity, a sure sign either of rupture of the bladder or of the renal pelvis. When performing a cystogram it is important to instill sufficient dye without pressure (usually a volume of 200 to 250 ml.) in order to get adequate filling and distention of the bladder; otherwise small lacerations can easily be missed. Lateral as well as anteroposterior projections must be obtained. Many ruptures of the bladder can be controlled adequately by perivesical drainage and transurethral catheterization, although surgical closure of the wound is preferable. If there is no necrotic tissue, urinary fistula formation from a ruptured bladder treated in this way rarely occurs. The uterus seldom is injured by trauma because it is so mobile. The same is true of the ovaries and tubes, since they are relatively mobile and adherent to the lateral wall of the pelvis; it is rather unusual for them to be damaged.

RETROPERITONEAL VASCULAR INJURIES SECONDARY TO TRAUMA

These include injuries of the abdominal aorta, inferior vena cava, the iliac arteries or veins and their branches, and the gonadal and lumbar vessels. A pelvic fracture often may be associated with massive retroperitoneal bleeding requiring 10 to 15 units of blood in rapid succession. It is difficult to ascertain whether such a pelvic fracture is associated with bleeding only from the highly vascular bone or from puncture of one of the pelvic wall vessels. The surgeon must be guided by the rate of bleeding, the appearance of any blood within the free peritoneal cavity, the general status of the patient, and the associated injuries. Examination of the pulses in the thigh may be helpful but often gives no clue to whether there is any major vascular injury. Development of a palpable mass usually indicates that there is bleeding from the bone, not just from the bony surface. Distribution of pain may indicate that there is nerve as well as vascular injury from the bony spicules. When serious blood loss continues, pelvic exploration should be carried out for fractures. If no specific vascular injury is detected, therapeutic ligation of both hypogastric arteries may control blood loss from massive pelvic fractures.

Injury to the aorta and its major anterior branches, the superior mesenteric artery, the celiac axis, and the inferior mesenteric artery, or to the inferior vena cava with its major lumbar tributaries and the common iliac veins is not very common with blunt trauma or shock wave concussion, but either may be a frequent occurrence from gunshot or stab wounds. Many of these patients never reach the care of a physician or get to an emergency ward before exsanguination, but some of these injuries are bruising wounds of these vessels that later go on to rupture. Others are of the type that damages one of the branches of a major vessel at its junction with the larger vessel, with temporary occlusion at any of these sites. It is particularly for such wounds as this that massive infusions of blood, through at least two cutdowns, may give a chance for the patient to be brought to the operating room, where with proper facilities survival may be possible. For any large open wound, caused by any sort of missile, insertion of a large pack is certainly the wisest procedure until adequate arrangements and technical assistance can be obtained. With any injury of the lower aorta, compression by the fist over a pack, even on the outside of the abdomen, may sufficiently occlude the aorta to permit adequate coronary and cerebral circulation until sufficient transfusion can be obtained. This may permit successful operative intervention in such a dire emergency. With massive bleeding through any abdominal wound the great tendency is to try to control the bleeding point directly with some sort of hemostatic instrument, but this usually fails and the use of a blunt pressure pack is to much greater avail.

ACUTE ABDOMINAL INFLAMMATORY DISEASE

SECTION 3

SOME GENERALIZATIONS

10

A broad classification of inflammatory diseases of the abdomen consists of those associated with perforation of the involved viscus and localized or generalized peritonitis and those that are nonperforative in nature. This latter group includes all the nonoperative types of acute inflammatory reactions and many related medical problems with abdominal manifestations. Since many inflammatory reactions in the peritoneal cavity go on to perforation, the physician's primary decision is whether or not an exploratory operation is required either to prevent perforation or because perforation has already occurred.

NONPERFORATIVE PROBLEMS OF AN INFLAMMATORY NATURE

Most acute inflammatory reactions in the peritoneal cavity require specific surgical treatment, but by no means is the diagnosis as clear-cut as it is with the perforative lesions. There are conditions for which surgical exploration is not indicated unless initial medical therapy fails to control the problem. These include acute pancreatitis, regional enteritis, primary peritonitis, acute diverticulitis, ulcerative colitis, gastroenteritis, acute peptic ulcer, renal infarction, cecal ulcer, pneumonia, and mesenteric adenitis. Whereas the differential diagnosis of various types of obstructive lesions of the small intestine may be difficult and often academic, the specific diagnosis in nonperforated inflammatory lesions is extremely important and can usually be arrived at by detailed attention to the history, the physical examination, and the laboratory aids.

The history is extremely important, since many patients with these conditions have had previous attacks with special characteristics that help to distinguish one disease process from another. The initial localization of pain, the timing of onset in relation to intake of food, the radiation of pain, the specific laboratory findings in the serum, or the x-ray examinations may be the key to the diagnosis. With this type of lesion more than any of the others described in this book, there is a certain period of time available to the surgeon to make a diagnosis. Many of the subtleties of clinical medicine can be brought to bear in these inflammatory lesions that produce acute abdominal processes.

PERFORATED INFLAMMATORY LESIONS

When inflammatory lesions perforate, a far more dangerous situation exists for the patient. The peritoneal cavity will tolerate a single episode of contamination, which if corrected rapidly will leave virtually no residual damage. When continuous soilage occurs, as it does from an untreated perforated viscus, this cannot be dealt with efficiently. Abscess formation, progressive and massive plasma volume deficit, absorption of toxic products, necrosis with severe metabolic acidosis, thrombocytopenia of sepsis, renal and hepatic failure, and eventual death will ensue.

The perforated lesion that is not detected early is responsible for the persistent mortality from such diseases as appendicitis, cholecystitis, diverticulitis, ulcer, and strangulated bowel obstruction. It is the physician's responsibility to identify and treat the acute inflammatory lesions, which may go on to perforation, either before perforation has occurred or soon enough after so that no permanent damage will result.

The management of the patient with a perforated viscus requires a twofold approach. There is no question about the need for surgical exploration; this is the prime consideration. It is vital, however, to choose the time for surgical exploration when the patient can best tolerate it. Although operative procedure should not be delayed, adequate hours should be taken to rehydrate the patient, replace deficient volume of blood and plasma, and correct, if possible, congestive failure and airway difficulties so that the operation can be performed with greater safety. Frequently the operation itself, draining infected peritoneal fluid, decompressing the diaphragms, and sealing the offending perforation, is the only way to restore the patient to adequate homeostasis.

ABDOMINAL LESIONS THAT MAY PERFORATE

11 ▬▬▬▬▬▬▬▬▬▬▬▬▬▬▬▬▬▬▬▬

ACUTE APPENDICITIS

Acute appendicitis is the most common inflammatory lesion within the abdominal cavity, and it can mimic almost any other lesion. It is the condition that should be thought of first when a patient presents with abdominal pain.

Despite its being so common, little is known about the etiology of acute appendicitis. It is believed that a mucosal lesion is the initiating factor, followed by a penetrating inflammatory process that by its own progression leads to inadequate blood supply of the appendiceal diverticulum and eventually to gangrene and perforation. The disease progresses much more rapidly in young children and in the elderly. The presence of a fecalith helps to explain the etiology as being on some sort of obstructive basis, and also increases the rapidity of the perforative process (Figure 3–11). Obstruction is produced distal to the fecalith and there is a direct erosive action of the fecalith on the inflamed bowel.

Although chronic appendicitis is certainly not a very common or accepted finding, it is not at all rare for patients to complain of similar attacks 6 months, a year, or longer previously that subsided spontaneously. Many patients who have their appendix removed as an incidental procedure during some other abdominal operation have a scarred appendix that obviously has been the seat of some sort of inflammatory reaction in the past.

Careful combination of the history, physical examination, and laboratory data may help produce the diagnosis in the "typical case" of appendicitis. Of the three, however, the findings on physical examination far outweigh either the laboratory data or the historical situation in any specific patient and are more likely to tip the surgeon's hand than anything else. In each instance of acute appendicitis, the location of the inflamed portion of the appendix in retrospect can usually account for whatever sequence of history or physical findings was present earlier. The findings vary greatly depending on whether or not the inflamed tip of the appendix lies deep in the pelvis, up against the anterior parietal peritoneum, retrocecally, or buried in a big wad of omentum. The position of the appendix may vary (Figure 11–1). It is really this great variability in the actual location of the inflamed and offending part that accounts for the tremendous variation in physical and historical findings in acute appendicitis.

The patient with acute appendicitis may complain of periumbilical pain that, after several hours, becomes localized to the right lower quadrant of the abdomen or toward the flank, even down into the pelvis. The patient may have nausea, crampy pain in the abdomen, or constipation, although occasionally he or she complains of

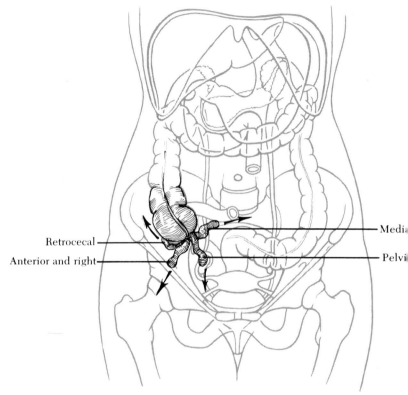

FIGURE 11–1 The vermiform appendix may vary greatly in its location.

some diarrhea. Anorexia is frequently a reliable symptom and may be of great value in differentiating appendicitis from many other temporary abdominal complaints. Usually when patients who were first observed with abdominal pain in the lower abdomen begin to regain their appetite, the likelihood of their having appendicitis becomes more remote. Sometimes, acute appendicitis may be preceded by attacks of upper abdominal pain, diarrhea, nausea, and vomiting, which may be typical of acute gastroenteritis, but as these subside the localized findings of appendicitis may begin.

The persistence of pain in the right lower quadrant cannot be overlooked or disregarded. Radiation down into the testicles or labia, or down into the thigh tends more to make one think of ureteral colic. In a woman pain typical of either mittelschmerz or menstrual pain can be produced by the appendix lying on the fallopian tube or the broad ligament. The pain of acute appendicitis may lack the usual referral phenomena if it is a true retrocecal appendix; that is, lying behind the peritoneal cavity retroperitoneally and retrocecally in the right flank. In this case the onset of pain usually begins at this locus and remains there. Contact with the anterior abdominal wall produces much more severe pain on coughing or motion of any sort and, of course, exquisite tenderness on examination.

As the inflammation of the appendix progresses the pain becomes more severe and the patient may develop chills, fever, and signs of toxicity. There may be a period of time just before perforation or at the time of perforation when the symptoms actually temporarily subside. This free interval occurring just prior to perforation when the patient seemingly gets somewhat better may delude the surgeon into delaying operation.

The physical examination is the most important part of the approach to the patient with acute abdominal disease, particularly in acute appendicitis. When the disease is actively progressing the patient wants to lie still in bed with the knees drawn up because any motion tends to produce more peritoneal irritation in the right lower quadrant. Light percussion often may localize the disease process without producing so much generalized pain that the patient is unable to aid in accurate identification of the area of tenderness. By this technique it may be possible to localize the tenderness to a square inch or so, often over McBurney's point.* The extent of peritoneal reaction determines the amount of spasm, both voluntary and involuntary, of the rectus abdominus and oblique musculature and the degree of rebound tenderness and its distribution. Rectal and pelvic tenderness also depend on the actual locus of the inflamed part. A positive psoas sign and positive obturator sign are determined by whether the inflamed appendix is posteriorly placed or not. Since it frequently lies posteriorly, these clinical signs are often positive in acute appendicitis. Pain with motion of the uterus can occur if the appendix lies against the tube or broad ligament; thus, differentiation between acute pelvic inflammatory disease and acute appendicitis may be difficult. Hyperesthesia of the right lower quadrant or even the right side of the abdomen may be noted in response to the irritated afferent pathway of the spinal nerve arc when the parietal peritoneum is inflamed.

In the absence of perforation of the appendix it is rare for the temperature to be above 101° F. in the adult, and it usually ranges between 99 and 100° F. Children and elderly persons may have more fever; in these patients peritonitis occurs more rapidly because there is poor lim-

*An arbitrary point two-thirds of the distance from the umbilicus to the anterior superior spine.

itation by the omentum and the blood supply has different characteristics.

The white blood cell count and the differential count are the most helpful laboratory studies available. Typically, in appendicitis, the white cell count is in the range of 11,000 to 15,000 per cubic millimeter with a shift to the left in band forms on the differential smear. Failure of a patient to develop leukocytosis or even an alteration in the differential count is not inconsistent with the diagnosis of acute appendicitis. The white cell count may be high when the patient is first seen with early symptoms and may slowly subside despite the progressive activity of acute appendicitis, or it may abruptly rise with no good correlation with the clinical findings. When the laboratory findings support those of the examination of the patient they can be valuable; when they fail to, the physical examination is most important.

Urinalysis is necessary to rule out any urinary tract disease, particularly ureteral lithiasis as indicated by hematuria. An inflamed appendix lying on the ureter may cause red cells and white cells to be present in the urine to further confuse the issue.

The sedimentation rate usually is elevated, but this is a difficult sign to follow unless one has been obtaining serial measurements. The hematocrit may not show much change unless perforation occurs, when its sharp elevation may reveal acute volume depletion due to plasma loss into the peritoneal cavity. The x-ray examination is primarily valuable in ruling out other causes of abdominal pain, although a fecalith can be identified in the right lower quadrant (Figure 3–11).

The diagnosis of acute appendicitis can be one of the easiest or one of the most difficult for a surgeon to make regardless of his or her experience. A high index of suspicion, a desire to observe the patient carefully over a period of hours, and a willingness to operate when and if physical signs and laboratory data continue to point toward acute appendicitis are essential. Usually 12 to 24 hours are available for careful repeated evaluation. The persistence of point tenderness must not be overlooked. It may be the only indication for surgical exploration.

The operative approach to appendicitis depends on the certainty of the diagnosis, the sex of the individual, and the localization of the positive findings. In a man, if the diagnosis is quite evident and the localized tenderness is in the most typical area, a muscle splitting incision, as described by McBurney or Rockie, is ideal and offers adequate exposure and excellent healing. If the diagnosis is in question, a rectus retracting incision is much wiser because wider exposure of the abdomen is possible. In a young woman, particularly of childbearing age, a right paramedian incision is more desirable because better evaluation of the pelvic organs can be made if the diagnosis of appendicitis is incorrect. Whenever possible, appendectomy should be carried out for acute appendicitis even if perforation or abscess formation has occurred as long as any localization about a previously perforated appendix is not disturbed.

The most common site of infection following appendectomy is the subcutaneous tissue in which contamination is frequent during surgery and the blood supply is usually poorest. For this reason either delayed primary closure or subcutaneous drains are often indicated. Other more serious complications of acute appendicitis are abscesses in the pelvis, the lateral gutter, or beneath the diaphragm, but most of these occur after perforation has occurred. Pylephlebitis is fortunately a rare complication in the present surgical era, but its association with hepatic abscesses still carries extremely high mortality.

PERFORATION IN APPENDICITIS

The length of time required for an acutely inflamed appendix to become gangrenous and then to perforate is dependent on several factors. In the very young or the very old patient, perforation tends to occur more rapidly, possibly owing to altered blood supply or to the status of the lymphoid tissue within the appendix. The presence of a fecalith within the appendix will make perforation much more rapid because it both provides a point of pressure, which erodes through the inflamed appendix, and produces obstruction and strangulation much more rapidly. Perforation occurs earlier in patients with diabetic and other types of vascular lesions. Free perforations are much more common in young children in whom the amount of omentum is small and there is very little attempt at walling-off the inflammatory reaction prior to perforation. A walled-off abscess is usually found when the appendix perforates. Omentum and small bowel serve to localize the abscess. Many patients have a combination of both free perforation with peritonitis, at least through the lower abdomen, and a loculated collection around the appendix and in the other common sites as well (Figure 11–2).

Sometimes a patient who has progressive right lower quadrant pain and tenderness will have a short period, maybe an hour or less, of abatement of some of these symptoms just prior to the time that perforation occurs.

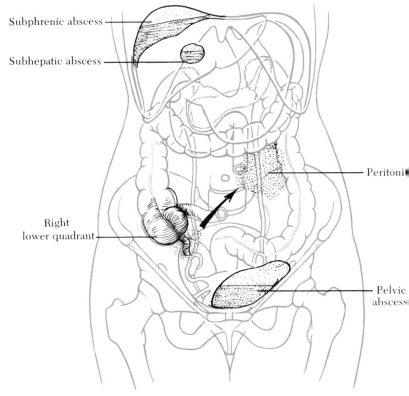

Subphrenic abscess

Subhepatic abscess

Peritoni

Right
lower quadrant

Pelvic
abscess

FIGURE 11–2 Locations of possible abscess formation from perforation in acute appendicitis.

Following this period in which both the patient and the physician may be lulled into a false sense of security, there will be the sudden onset of more severe lower abdominal and diffuse pain often associated with increased tachycardia, higher fever (usually 101° to 103°), and a more generally toxic appearance. The white count goes up into the 15,000 to 25,000/cu. mm. range; there is more tenderness in the cul-de-sac; peristalsis is absent; and there is more rebound, cough pain, and involuntary spasm and rigidity. Whereas rebound tenderness may have been localized to the area of the unperforated appendix, after perforation occurs there will be rebound tenderness referred from various places in the lower abdomen and even in the right upper quadrant to the right lower quadrant; indicating a much more diffuse peritonitis. Rarely is any free air seen on the plain or upright film of the abdomen in these patients.

The patient with acute appendicitis may develop a well walled-off abscess so that no free leak ever develops. He may present to the physician with a mass and a 4- or 5-day history of vague right lower quadrant pain. The walling-off probably occurred very early in the onset of the disease or even may have been present previously so that the degree of peritoneal signs and pain were reduced so much that the physician's services were not sought earlier. This mass often can be felt on bimanual examination, depending on how far into the pelvis it extends. Toxicity is much less apparent, but prompt surgical drainage is still indicated because these abscesses may be poorly bounded and free perforation can occur spontaneously. Rarely, such a patient will have spontaneous drainage and a fecal fistula will result.

If a walled-off abscess is encountered, the primary objective of a surgeon is to drain it adequately. Whenever possible, the appendix should be removed at the same time, if it can be identified and if the condition of the patient permits. Frequently the cecum can be identified and the appendix may be removed in a retrograde manner;

that is, by dividing the stump and turning it in first, and then dissecting down the mesentery until the entire appendix can be freed and removed. There may be occasions when the appendix may be left in place with wide drainage of the appendiceal abscess, and then a few months later an incidental appendectomy is performed. A barium enema should be considered prior to interval appendectomy, since a malignant lesion may be the basis for a more chronic inflammatory reaction in the appendix.

ACUTE CHOLECYSTITIS

Acute inflammatory processes in the right upper quadrant of the abdomen require differentiation among acute cholecystitis, acute pancreatitis, and acute peptic ulcer as well as gastroenteritis and hepatitis (Figure 11–3). Of these, the acute inflammation of the gallbladder may be the first symptom that the patient has ever had of gallbladder disease. Often, however, a history of previous attacks can be obtained. The typical picture of chronic cholecystitis is one of pain starting in the epigastrium or the right upper quadrant with radiation through to the back or to the base of the right scapula. Previous attacks of pain are rarely as severe as the attack that brings the patient to the hospital. Frequently a history of fatty food intolerance may be obtained; it is not unusual for such a patient to have actually had a previous gallbladder study that demonstrated stones on x-ray examination. A history of jaundice should always be sought. The possibility of recurrent chills and fever, severe crampy abdominal pain, and the other sequelae of biliary colic may be brought out. Nausea, vomiting, anorexia, and fairly steady epigas-

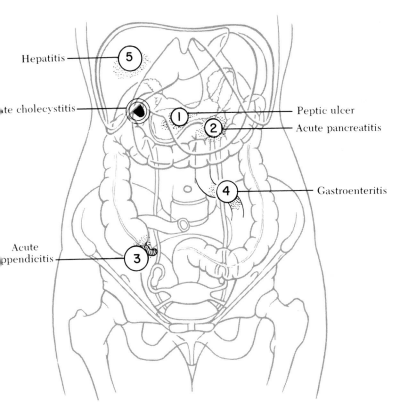

FIGURE 11–3   Considerations in the differential diagnosis of acute cholecystitis: 1, acute peptic ulcer; 2, acute pancreatitis; 3, acute appendicitis; 4, acute gastroenteritis; 5, hepatitis.

tric pain are the usual symptoms the patient complains of. This disease is more common in females, particularly after pregnancy. In the young woman a splenic hemolytic anemia must always be considered. There is a high incidence of cholecystitis in the elderly person as well, and here it is a much more dangerous disease than in the middle-aged woman. In the elderly, the gallbladder may become gangrenous much more quickly, it takes very little vomiting to dehydrate the patient, and many other systemic diseases may make primary surgical management more difficult.

On physical examination of the patient with acute cholecystitis, right upper quadrant tenderness is a fairly consistent finding and there may be associated hyperesthesia, spasm, voluntary guarding, and pain on deep inspiration. Of particular use is Murphy's sign, a forced splinting of the lower chest when the examiner palpates at the costal border as the patient inspires. This rarely is seen when an acute peptic ulcer is present. Liver tenderness also may be present; in most cases the gallbladder itself cannot be palpated because it lies beneath the liver edge and to a great extent within the liver bed. Sometimes, however, a large palpable tender gallbladder may be felt, particularly in cases of either empyema or hydrops of the gallbladder. A patient with recurring attacks of cholecystitis may have a scarred, thickened, contracted gallbladder that never becomes distended or palpable. In the case of the chronically inflamed gallbladder, or when cholecystitis is recurrent, the omentum may become adherent over the gallbladder, thus reducing its sensitivity.

The patient may be slightly icteric since acute cholecystitis even without the passage of common duct stones may be associated with a slightly elevated bilirubin, up to about 3 mg. per 100 ml. The presence of dark urine and light stools associated with symptoms of acute cholecystitis usually indicates common duct obstruction by stone disease rather than jaundice associated with acute cholecystitis alone. In addition to the bilirubin level in the serum, it is important to obtain a prothrombin time to be certain that underlying liver disease is not present and need not be corrected before surgery. The white blood cell count is usually elevated, but since acute cholecystitis begins as a chemical inflammation secondary to obstruction of the ampulla of the gallbladder, the white cell count may be normal in early cases of acute cholecystitis before any secondary infection supervenes. It is always important to determine the serum amylase level, since acute pancreatitis may be very difficult to differentiate from acute cholecystitis and may also be a concomitant disease.

Although localized right upper quadrant tenderness, spasm, and pain, and an excellent history indicative of biliary tract disease may be sufficient evidence to make a diagnosis of acute cholecystitis, the presence of either jaundice, a palpable gallbladder, or gallstones visualized either by plain films of the abdomen or an oral cholecystogram ideally should be confirmed to reach accurate diagnosis sufficient for performing an operation. It may be difficult to rule out the possibility of acute duodenal ulcer or acute pancreatitis by abdominal examination alone, although the varying features of these diseases are discussed later. High levels of serum amylase certainly suggest pancreatitis but cannot absolutely rule out cholecystitis as well. Patients with diabetes mellitus have a slightly higher incidence of acute cholecystitis than the general population, and these patients should be operated on much more quickly since gangrene of the gallbladder occurs with greater frequency.

The operative management of acute cholecystitis

should be cholecystectomy whenever possible. The surgeon should, on certain specific occasions, be willing to perform a cholecystostomy with the full realization that a later cholecystectomy may be necessary. For a cholecystostomy to be effective, adequate removal of all the obstructing gallstones must be carried out. In many cases of acute cholecystitis in which there is tremendous edema and swelling of the fundus and body of the gallbladder, the degree of reaction about the cystic artery and duct may be fairly minimal, permitting a safe cholecystectomy. Since the acute episode of cholecystitis often will subside after a few hours, the surgeon has two options: either proceed with cholecystectomy or schedule the operation as an elective procedure. The authors favor early operation. The concept of a waiting period or a period of antibiotic therapy generally has been discarded.

ACALCULOUS CHOLECYSTITIS

Acalculous cholecystitis, acute and chronic, constitutes only a small percentage of all instances of cholecystitis. The signs and symptoms are identical to those of calculous cholecystitis. However, the diagnosis of acalculous cholecystitis is difficult to confirm because most patients with the disease have normal cholecystograms, and surgeons understandably are reluctant to remove the gallbladder under these circumstances. Recently it has been pointed out that repeated delayed roentgenograms of the gallbladder after the initial examination may be helpful in the diagnosis of acalculous cholecystitis. In patients suspected clinically of having cholecystitis and whose oral cholecystograms are normal, delayed roentgenograms of the gallbladder are made 24 hours after the initial examination. Persistent opacification 36 hours after the ingestion of Telepaque strongly suggests that the gallbladder is diseased and that the patient does have acalculous cholecystitis. The management and treatment are the same as for calculous cholecystitis, except that exploration of the common duct may be necessary to rule out stones passed into the common bile duct.

BILIARY COLIC

Biliary colic may accompany acute cholecystitis or may be present in patients without any active inflammation of the gallbladder. In general, there is a past history similar to that of the patient with chronic recurrent cholecystitis; that is, fatty food intolerance, often with previous episodes of chills, fever, jaundice, and most of all sharp, crampy pain radiating through to the shoulder, back, or scapula that causes the patient to double up in agony. It is one of the most severe types of pain that patients complain of. If cholangitis is associated with the presence of common duct stone disease, then chills and fever accompany the complaints. The jaundice may occur rapidly and disappear just as rapidly if the patient passes a common duct stone. The passage of one stone, however, in no way negates the indication for surgical intervention since there are usually other stones present in the common duct or stones continually moving into the common duct from the gallbladder.

Biliary colic may be a sequela of previous gallbladder surgery in which the common duct was not explored and stones were left behind or else have formed *de novo.* The

possibility of stricture or common duct injury with subsequent stone formation must also be taken into account.
The presence of bile in the urine (detected by either the
Harrison spot test or the shake test), acholic stools, and
an elevated icteric index, serum bilirubin, and alkaline
phosphatase all add up to the chemical diagnosis of common duct stone disease. SGOT and LDH determinations
may be normal or slightly elevated, depending upon the
time course of the disease. Physical findings on examination may be minimal, particularly hepatic tenderness, but
as stated, acute cholecystitis may also be present. Stool
examination must always be carried out since the finding
of occult blood may signal the presence of an ampullary
carcinoma or a tumor of the head of the pancreas. A mild
rise in the serum amylase may occur even with common
duct stone disease without clinical pancreatitis.

In the jaundiced patient it is usually possible to differentiate between biliary colic and carcinoma obstructing the biliary tree when the jaundice is associated with
an acute, painful history. When hepatic obstruction due
to stone disease occurs as a much more subtle involvement, the diagnosis becomes much less certain. The
presence of a palpable, distended, nontender gallbladder
(Courvoisier), changes in the duodenal loop on an
upper GI series, evidence of malabsorption, weight loss,
anemia, or diabetes all may aid in arriving at a diagnosis
of carcinoma.

Exploration of the common duct need not be considered an emergency procedure in patients with common
duct obstruction due to stone disease. If the patient has
evidence of ascending cholangitis it becomes more
urgent to relieve the partially obstructed duct. Antibiotics
should be begun prior to surgery in these cases. It is most

important that the surgeon be thorough in his exploration and that he carefully identify both hepatic ducts as well as the distal common duct by probing and by common duct cholangiography. Retained stones in the upper tracts within the liver pose very serious problems in the long-term management of the patient. It is our policy to use T-tube drainage of the explored common duct and to obtain cholangiograms both at the time of operation and approximately 10 days following operation, prior to removal of the short-limbed T-tube.

ACUTE PEPTIC ULCER

Gastric and duodenal ulcer disease must be considered as a single entity since it is often impossible to distinguish between them in their acute forms. The acute ulcer may be the first evidence of ulcer disease for that patient or it may be part of a long-standing history. The pain of peptic ulcer may be very typical, occurring in the right upper quadrant or epigastrium, well localized, frequently radiating through to the back, exacerbated at night, and relieved by food and antacids in a nervous, tense person.

It is for complications of ulcer disease that patients usually present with acute abdominal problems. Obstruction, bleeding, perforation, and intractable pain all require immediate care (Figure 11–4). The patient with an acute but uncomplicated ulcer generally has localized tenderness in the right upper quadrant without any mass palpable. This pain may be more frequently associated with vomiting if the ulcer lies in the pyloric channel, although vomiting may accompany any acute ulcer. Gastric ulcers may be associated with more "indigestion" than

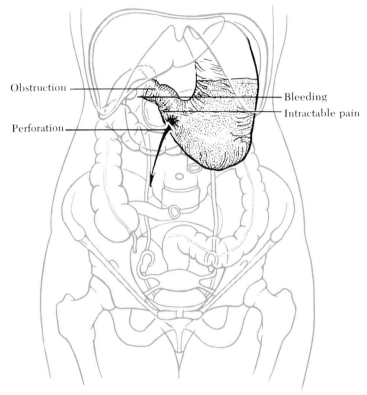

FIGURE 11–4 The complications of peptic ulcer that may require surgery.

duodenal ulcer disease, which produces less localized tenderness and more of a crampy element to the pain. In either gastric or duodenal ulcer disease the pain may be diffuse across the upper abdomen, but the tenderness may be well localized. Fever is not common and only a mild leukocytosis may be present. The diagnosis sometimes can be confirmed by finding either occult or gross blood in the stomach if nasogastric suction is instituted. Upper gastrointestinal x-rays should be obtained when the diagnosis is questionable. Acute peptic ulcers are best treated by very intense, around-the-clock treatment with sedation and gastric acid neutralization. Rapid relief of symptoms may occur with such therapy, and the need for surgical exploration can be eliminated if acute ulcers are treated before they perforate or penetrate into the surrounding tissues.

PERFORATED PEPTIC ULCER

For many patients with peptic ulcer disease, the first sign or symptom that they are aware of may be the acute perforation. Careful questioning of these patients may reveal that for a few days or even several weeks prior to the actual perforation some upper abdominal discomfort, often night pain, existed. Perforation of an ulcer often occurs after a meal or a bout of drinking when the stomach is distended. The pain at the time of perforation is knifelike and the patient can usually time it very accurately. From that point on it usually remains steady, sharp, and anterior since the perforations occur on the anterior part of stomach or duodenum. Occasionally a perforation is placed more posteriorly, draining into the lesser sac, and in these cases the pain is more bizarre, more posteriorly placed, and less well localized. The pain of perforated ulcer is severe and accompanied by immediate, diffuse peritoneal irritation with boardlike rigidity, rebound, spasm, and the full-blown picture of free perforation of a hollow viscus. The complication of ulcer disease usually occurs in younger people, more commonly in men than women, and the abdominal musculature is frequently so powerfully in spasm that it is impossible to discern much upon abdominal examination except that there is diffuse upper abdominal peritonitis.

The patient usually can localize the onset of tenderness to the right upper quadrant or epigastrium, but by the time he or she is examined, the pain is already diffuse, as are the findings. Vomiting may contain blood because erosion precedes the perforation and the mucosa may have bled at the time. Massive bleeding rarely accompanies a perforated ulcer. The serum amylase may be elevated with any perforation of the upper intestinal tract, usually as a result of resorption of the enzymes from the peritoneal cavity. The finding of benzidine-positive material in the vomitus or by aspiration of the stomach may help to differentiate this lesion from that of acute pancreatitis, which may also have a sudden onset with very severe signs. Acute gastritis can, however, accompany acute pancreatitis.

When a patient with acute perforation of a peptic ulcer is first seen by the physician the severity of pain is usually the most impressive finding. There is a rapid plasma volume deficit due to the chemical peritonitis from the acidic gastric contents; hypotension and tachycardia often may be present, and the use of narcotics for pain relief may be dangerous. Fluid therapy, both plasma and saline, should be begun immediately to restore the volume deficit while any necessary investigation of the patient is performed.

X-ray examination of the abdomen and chest by plain film and upright or lateral decubitus x-rays may often demonstrate free air beneath the diaphragm or in the peritoneal cavity. About 75 per cent of the patients with perforated duodenal or gastric ulcers show such free air to be present on initial x-rays. Upright or decubitus films must be taken after the patient has had sufficient time in that position for any air within the peritoneal cavity to accumulate beneath the diaphragm. Rarely, especially with a posterior perforation, a barium swallow or Gastrografin swallow may be indicated when the diagnosis is strongly suspected but cannot be substantiated by the usual physical and x-ray procedures (Chapter Three).

The LDH level may be elevated as well as the hematocrit. Leukocytosis is usually present but may still be normal when the patient is first seen. The serum amylase level may be mildly elevated, possibly two or even three times normal at the maximum. If the ulcer penetrates posteriorly and then perforates, a greater degree of pancreatitis may be present.

Surgical control of the perforated ulcer is definitely the treatment of choice. It can never be predicted when, even with constant gastric suction, such a perforated ulcer will become spontaneously sealed. Even the acutely ill patient can have an operation carried out under local anesthesia or very light general anesthesia supplementing local anesthesia, and have a swift, yet adequate, plication of the ulcer with omentum. If perforated ulcers simply are closed within a period of 12 to 18 hours after the onset of perforation, prompt recovery is the rule since the peritoneum will withstand this degree of trauma well. As much as possible of the spilled gastric contents should be evacuated and if free distribution has already occurred, then irrigation into the peritoneal gutters, around the liver, and under the diaphragm will help. If the ulcer appears to be in the stomach rather than the duodenum a biopsy should always be carried out to be certain that this is not a carcinoma, but duodenal ulcers do not require biopsy.

There is no way that perforation from a previously undiagnosed gastric carcinoma can be distinguished preoperatively unless the age of the patient and a history of debilitation provide clues. Abdominal exploration is still necessary, even if only for palliative therapy. Approximately one-third of the patients who have perforated ulcer as their primary symptom of peptic ulcer disease will never have any further difficulty with this disease on conservative therapy once the plication has been carried out. Another third will eventually come to surgery because of complications of their ulcer disease, and the final third will have some symptoms not severe enough to require surgical management. With newer and less disabling surgical approaches to the management of ulcer disease, such as the use of pyloroplasty and vagotomy, it is possible that a greater number of these patients will subsequently have surgical procedures performed for their ulcer disease.

DIVERTICULITIS

Inflammatory lesions may occur throughout the colon (Figure 11–5), but diverticulitis is the most common. Acute diverticulitis usually occurs in the sigmoid or the left colon. Although the patient may have diverticula throughout the large intestine, the disease of diverticulitis is usually localized to a few inches of the colon. Diverticulitis begins as many microabscesses in the wall

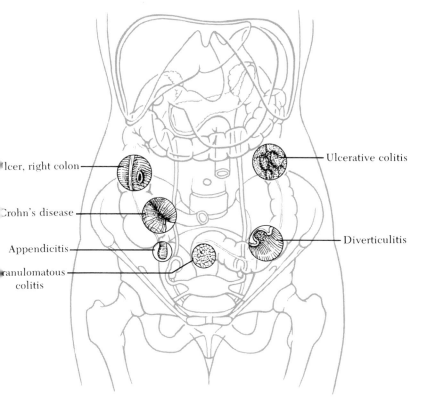

Ulcer, right colon

Crohn's disease

Appendicitis

Granulomatous colitis

Ulcerative colitis

Diverticulitis

FIGURE 11–5   Examples of inflammatory lesions of the large bowel.

of the colon with the inflammatory reaction extending through the wall in the area of the diverticulum. Once initiated, it involves the entire wall of the colon. There is a great deal of induration and thickening of the bowel at the site of the diverticulitis. It never is initiated below the pelvic peritoneal floor. Gross intramural and pericolic abscesses frequently develop as the disease progresses. It is important to understand the pathologic entity of diverticulitis in order to appreciate the disease and its pathogenesis.

Pain is the foremost symptom of diverticulitis; it is usually in the left lower quadrant or left-sided, depending on the exact site of the inflammatory mass. Although constipation and some evidence of low-grade obstruction are the usual results of the inflammatory thickening and narrowing of the wall of the colon, occasionally diarrhea may be the presenting finding, possibly related to partial obstruction or localized irritation and hypermobility. Bleeding may occur in a significant number of cases, and massive bleeding may be present in as many as 10 per cent of cases of diverticulitis. Occult bleeding is present in many more since this is a mucosal lesion in part. When the presenting lesion is a large inflammatory area, then fever, chills, tenderness, and a palpable mass all make themselves apparent.

Occasionally, massive bleeding or one of the other complications of diverticulitis (Figure 11–6) is the initial way in which this disease presents itself; and these will be discussed in subsequent sections. The usual method of presentation is with pain due to acute inflammatory reaction before any perforation, massive bleeding, or obstruction has occurred. Local fistulization, especially to the bladder, is a frequent consequence of diverticulitis but is rarely the presenting finding. There is usually a chronic history of lower abdominal pains and some cramps with a more acute inflammatory reaction developing as more of an intramural and extramural abscess, or at least inflammatory mass, develops. To separate this disease into any one of its complicating lesions

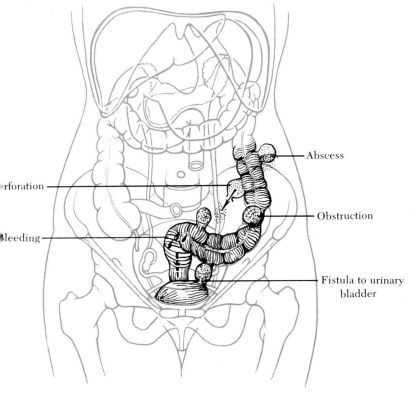

FIGURE 11–6 Complications of diverticulitis.

would be an error. The major symptoms and problems with diverticulitis are presented in this section and the other complications are included in the various other sections.

When a patient presents with a history of lower abdominal crampy pain, particularly on the left, diverticulitis must be a prime diagnosis regardless of the age of the patient. Diverticulitis used to be considered a disease of the aged, but, in fact, this disease is not at all rare in the third and fourth decades.

The sigmoid colon is most frequently involved, but occasionally a redundant sigmoid lies on the right side of the abdomen, producing a clinical picture of diverticulitis indistinguishable from acute appendicitis. The lower abdominal pain may be steady, but is usually crampy and accompanied by fever and chills, depending on whether or not pus is present in an abscess. Chronic constipation is usual, but occasionally diarrhea is present, particularly tenesmus with a distal sigmoid lesion.

Examination reveals localized tenderness in the left lower quadrant; generally, there is some ileus. There may be enough obstruction to produce hyperactive and high-pitched peristaltic sounds and even some reflex vomiting. A mass may be palpable in the sigmoid by abdominal examination in the left lower quadrant just above the brim of the pelvis. When the disease is higher in the left colon it is very difficult to feel a mass, but there may be localized tenderness. The left colon is more deeply placed here and protected by the kidney posteriorly and the omentum anteriorly. Occasionally a mass can be felt in the flank, which represents left colonic diverticulitis, particularly if an abscess has formed. By rectal or pelvic examination the sigmoid mass may sometimes be palpated. It is more often at the brim of the pelvis rather than in the true pelvis and is best palpated abdominally.

The extent of physical findings is proportional to the severity of the inflammatory reaction. There may be just thickened, inflamed bowel, or there may be a large walled-off pelvic abscess with diffuse pelvic peritonitis.

Since diverticulitis really consists of small perforations of the colon, it is easy to realize that abscess formation is just a direct extension of the basic disease. The stool should always be checked for occult blood, since about one-third of patients with diverticulitis have occult blood in their stool. Diverticulitis may coexist with cancer, although there is no evidence that it predisposes to malignancy.

The white blood cell count usually is elevated with the inflammatory reaction and may be a good gauge of the response to conservative management. Sigmoidoscopy always should be carried out both to identify the inflammatory lesion, which is often present at about 15 to 20 cm. from the anus, and to attempt to get a tissue diagnosis to rule out the possibility of coexistent carcinoma. A barium enema gently done may be of great value in making a diagnosis in the acute case of diverticulitis (Chapter Three). The combination of barium enema studies, stool smears for malignant cells by the Papanicolaou technique, and sigmoidoscopy or colonoscopy is the method for preoperative differentiation between carcinoma and simple diverticulitis. Frequently, the patient has had documentation of diverticulitis by previous barium enema studies, and the disease, previously treated by conservative management, may present with an acute exacerbation.

The last 20 years has seen a marked change in the treatment of diverticulitis. This disease was considered to be an inevitable successor to diverticulosis, and it was the consensus that minimal surgical therapy should be instituted unless complications ensued. More active treatment at any earlier stage has become common. Treatment for the complications requires a two- or three-stage procedure stretched out over many months. More aggressive therapy dictates conservative management of the initial lesion to see whether it will subside adequately to permit a one-stage resection of the colon as an elective procedure after the first major episode of diverticulitis. This has permitted more satisfactory and effective treatment for cure of this disease. If the patient has a large inflammatory abscess, one usually reverts to the three-stage procedure with colostomy in the right transverse colon and drainage of the abscess as the initial step. If no true abscess has developed and the lesion can be resected, primary resection and anastomosis with or without complementary diversion of the fecal stream proximal to the anastomosis may be the treatment of choice. Another excellent operative approach, when mesenteric length permits, is exteriorization and resection of the involved segment of sigmoid with subsequent closure of the double-barreled sigmoid colostomy. Considerable judgment must be exercised by the surgeon to choose the proper procedure for the individual patient. Antibiotic therapy, bed rest, and intestinal preparation with nonabsorbable sulfa and Neomycin are instituted when the acute inflammatory lesion presents — unless it is obvious that immediate drainage of an abscess is essential.

PERFORATION IN DIVERTICULITIS

It is uncommon for the initial bout of diverticulitis to be one of free perforation of the colon. When perforation occurs, either an abscess adjacent to the site of perforation develops, if sufficient inflammatory walling-off has occurred, or generalized peritonitis results. It is entirely possible for a large pelvic abscess to be the first symptom of diverticular disease, since this may build up over a period of several days as the pericolonic extension of disease fails to form a well-localized mass. Fistula formation is usually a delayed consequence and rarely presents as an acute problem.

The history of a patient with freely perforating diverticulitis is again the rather acute onset of sharp, steady pain in the area of the diverticulitis. This is usually the left lower quadrant and, because there is immediate onset of peritoneal irritation, this pain and these findings do not begin periumbilically but rather as an immediate, localized pain at the site of perforation. The degree of peritoneal soilage determines the extent of the rebound, distention, spasm, and local tenderness. Ileus is the rule, and the patient is usually more toxic than with upper abdominal and small bowel perforations. In general, perforations of the large bowel are more lethal than other intestinal perforations.

Occasionally the first sign of perforation is evidence of a fistula formation or perforation into the bladder, more common in the male or in the female after hysterectomy. The patient complains of pneumaturia and feculent urine, this really being a type of fistula rather than any free perforation. By rectal and bimanual examination a mass may often be felt in the pelvis, particularly in the case of the large pelvic abscess related to a walled-off perforation of diverticulitis. Large and small bowel obstruction may be related to such an abscess as well as to a severe degree of paralytic ileus. The stool may occasionally be benzidine-positive, but those cases of diverticulitis that perforate rarely have any significant degree of bleeding. Sigmoidoscopy should always be the initial step because it is never possible to be certain whether or not diverticulitis or carcinoma or both are present when patients present with these findings. It is very difficult at the time of surgery to be certain which problem one is dealing with, and therefore any information that can be obtained by intraluminal evaluation through the sigmoidoscope, either preoperatively or intraoperatively, is always of great value.

Diverticulitis of the cecum and transverse colon, which are often solitary, can perforate and mimic carcinoma entirely in these loci; there is no recourse but to treat them as carcinoma with fairly extensive resection. The management of perforated diverticulitis and perforated carcinoma is entirely different when the diagnosis can be differentiated; this is the reason for trying to make the differentiation.

Emergency barium enema is also extremely helpful. This should be performed under absolutely no pressure with very careful cooperation between the fluoroscopist and the surgeon. If the fluoroscopist can demonstrate a site of perforation, he or she should immediately cease any further study.

When diverticulitis is the cause of such colonic perforation, the primary aim of the surgeon is to divert the fecal stream; a right transverse colostomy is the procedure of choice with adequate drainage in the area of the perforation, particularly if a walled-off abscess has formed. If a free perforation exists in a localized lesion, an alternate procedure is to carry out local primary resection and anastomosis.

Prolonged ileus often follows a perforation, even when a colostomy has been performed. Nasogastric suction, careful attention to fluid and electrolyte replacement, and maintenance of adequate intravascular volume are essential in these patients.

ULCERATIVE COLITIS

Ulcerative colitis, much like regional enteritis and diverticulitis, is a disease that is usually chronic with frequent exacerbations, any one of which may be acute enough to make the patient present to the surgeon with an acutely inflamed abdomen. The initial attack may be

TABLE 11–1   Inflammatory Diseases of the Colon

	Ulcerative Colitis	Granulomatous Colitis	Diverticulitis
Usual location	Rectum, left colon, entire colon	Right colon, ileum	Sigmoid (98%)
Rectal involvement	Nearly all patients	About 20% of patients	None
Rectal bleeding	Common, continuous	Less common, intermittent	Frequent, usually occult
Fistulas	Rare	Common	Frequent, especially to urinary bladder
Bowel stricture	Rare	Common	Narrowing usually due to spasm
Toxic megacolon	Frequent	Rare	None
Perforation	Frequent	Rare	Common
Carcinoma	Common in chronic states	Rare	Rare

sufficiently acute to appear as a solitary abdominal situation. As with diverticulitis there are many different forms that this disease can take, and there are numerous complications, any of which may be reason enough for surgical management. Contrary to that for diverticulitis, the surgical management of the acute disease is limited to the complications; whenever possible, conservative medical management should be attempted for ulcerative colitis.

This disease usually occurs in the young age group. The patient may have as many as 10 to 15 bloody stools a day accompanied by mucus, cramps, tenesmus, debility, and weight loss. Acute fever, diarrhea, and pain may, however, be the initial method of presentation. A diagnosis of ulcerative colitis should be suspected when a young patient has bloody mucus with diarrhea. Ulcerative colitis may begin on the right side of the colon and remain there for several years before becoming diffuse. This type may be much more difficult to diagnose at an early stage, but the barium enema can be of great value. Most commonly, the disease develops in the rectum, the sigmoid, and the left colon; it may not involve the right side at all. The right-sided disease, of course, may be confused with acute appendicitis, but there is frequently associated bleeding to help separate the two. Regional enteritis and ulcerative colitis may be very closely related and, in fact, regional enteritis may involve the colon in the form of ileocolitis, whereas ulcerative colitis less commonly involves the small intestine.

The acutely inflamed bowel may be tender and boggy, and produce typical right lower quadrant or left lower quadrant masses, which can be confused with other types of lesions. Sigmoidoscopy will help greatly in differentiating this diagnosis because even though a mass may be present in the high sigmoid by physical examination, the ulcerative disease usually involves the rectum and the distal sigmoid. The typical shallow granular ulcers with ragged mucosa between them and the excoriation and thickening of pseudopolyps may be identified and biopsy specimens taken on sigmoidoscopic examination.

The best treatment for this disease at the present time is conservative management with diet, rest, nonabsorbable antibiotics, topical and systemic steroid therapy, and supportive measures such as blood transfusions, fluids, and sedation.

Colonic perforation in ulcerative colitis is a grave consequence. A patient with known ulcerative colitis who has been stable on medical therapy may suddenly have exacerbation of the disease with multiple sites of perforation due to invasive sepsis of the bowel. Such a patient is extremely ill, has severe tachycardia, fever, and septicemia. Acute desalting water loss and major colloid deficit are superimposed upon chronic illness. Frequently, perforation in ulcerative colitis is a result of the large bowel just "falling apart," and there is little if any attempt at walling-off of the perforated site or sites. If the diagnosis has not been noted previously, sigmoidoscopy is essential to confirm it. The usual abdominal signs of generalized peritonitis are quickly apparent in such patients. The surgical treatment is an emergency ileostomy with total abdominoperineal resection of the colon and rectum, even though the patient appears to be in dire condition. Massive bleeding may also accompany perforation in such cases, making the need for colectomy even more urgent. Repeated seeding of the portal venous system with bacteria may be the major cause of mortality here.

REGIONAL ENTERITIS

Regional enteritis or ileitis may present to the surgeon as an acute or chronic inflammatory lesion of the small intestine, often discovered at the time of operation for some other problem. When acute regional enteritis involves the distal ileum, there is very little about it to distinguish it from acute appendicitis by history or physical examination unless have been premonitory signs, evidence of chronic disease, diarrhea, bloody stool, obstruction, and weight loss. Unfortunately, even the presence of known regional enteritis will not be sufficient to prevent exploration of the abdomen if everything points to acute appendicitis and the appendix is still in place. On several occasions patients with known regional enteritis of a chronic nature have had acute appendicitis superimposed as a separate disease.

X-ray examination is not carried out in the acute situation, but if the symptoms begin to subside under close observation, then a barium enema and an upper GI series may be done.

Free perforation is rare; fistula, obstruction, and abscess formation are more common. With the development of an abscess, drainage is essential if it is large. Small abscesses within the loops of the bowel and fistula formation should be treated in a very conservative manner. If the disease is localized with a fistula or perforation, local resection can be carried out, but a rigidly conservative approach appears safest.

Controversy still exists as to whether, when a patient undergoes an exploratory operation for acute right lower quadrant pain and is found to have regional enteritis of the ileum not involving the cecum, the appendix should be removed to avoid the necessity of later operation. The policy of the authors is to remove the appendix under these circumstances unless the cecum and the base of the appendix are involved with regional enteritis.

MECKEL'S DIVERTICULUM

It is impossible to differentiate acute Meckel's diverticulitis from acute appendicitis except when ectopic gastric mucosa is present within the lumen of the Meckel's diverticulum. Under those circumstances, bleeding into the lumen of the gut may occur secondary to the inflammation with resultant blood in the stool. A previous history compatible with intussusception may give a lead to the possibility of a Meckel's diverticulum being present, although that is unusual. The onset of pain localized in the right lower quadrant with local peritoneal signs is typical of Meckel's diverticulitis. It is so much more rare than acute appendicitis that little differentiation need be done except that abdominal exploration is necessary. Whenever an exploratory operation for acute appendicitis is performed and the acute appendix is not found, the small intestine should always be examined carefully for the presence of a Meckel's diverticulum located about two feet proximal to the ileocecal valve.

Perforation of the Meckel's diverticulum may occur much more rapidly than in acute appendicitis, especially if active gastric mucosa is present. The possibility of carcinoid tumors within the Meckel's diverticulum is real, and the liver should always be carefully examined for the presence of any metastasis when a Meckel's diverticulum appears to have a mass in its tip. Resection of the diverticulum is the treatment of choice.

PERFORATION OF INTESTINAL CARCINOMA

SMALL INTESTINE

Small intestinal carcinomas are unusual lesions and rarely are the cause of free perforation. If the cancer extends through the wall of the bowel, the formation of a fistula to another loop of intestine is the usual result rather than free perforation. Small bowel perforations may occur from metastatic extension of tumor rising in other organs such as stomach, large intestine, ovary, and pancreas. When such small bowel lesions do produce free perforation a degree of intestinal obstruction often precedes this. Little specific information can be given about how to establish the diagnosis except that a generalized peritonitis ensues with the usual physical findings and surgical exploration is indicated. Sometimes local abscess formation results when perforations occur that do not form fistulas.

LARGE INTESTINE

Free perforation, abscess formation locally, or fistulas are possible when large intestinal carcinomas perforate. Of these, abscess and fistula formation are the most common, as with small intestinal lesions. Carcinoma of the large intestine is much more common, and perforative lesions occur more frequently. An obstructive element is often present, possibly identified only in retrospect, before perforation occurs. A history of crampy abdominal pain with changes in the bowel habits before the onset of severe abdominal pain may be elicited. The patient seen with a perforated carcinoma has local and generalized peritoneal signs and is usually ill with fever, tachycardia, diffuse rebound tenderness, distention, spasm, and absence of peristalsis. The stool is often positive for occult blood.

Whereas for diverticulitis of the colon with perforation drainage and diversion are the treatment of choice, in the case of carcinoma, resection of the lesion responsible for the perforation should be attempted. Sigmoidoscopy should be carried out in an attempt to identify a low-lying lesion so that the proper approach can be planned. The best survival results in patients with perforated carcinoma are obtained with primary resection and anastomosis, and diverting colostomy if necessary A second best to resection and anastomosis is the defunctionalizing colostomy or a bypass procedure with early resection when the patient's condition warrants it. The Mikulicz resection has an occasional place in the treatment of perforated carcinoma of the sigmoid.

STRANGULATION NECROSIS OF THE INTESTINE

Small intestine lesions that are responsible for strangulation as a consequence of obstruction are adhesive bands, hernias (both internal and external), volvulus, intussusception, and congenital malformation. The congenital malformations include duplications of the intestinal tract. In the large intestine, volvulus is the major lesion responsible, but hernia, particularly incisional and inguinal hernias, may also lead to strangulation and obstruction.

All these underlying conditions except, possibly,

duplication of the small intestine usually are preceded by intestinal obstruction that persists for a period of days, or at least hours, as the proximal obstructed bowel becomes more edematous, develops capillary and venous occlusion caused by the obstructing condition, and eventually arterial obstruction and gangrenous perforation. All these patients have serious metabolic derangements. They have been undergoing major shifts in plasma volume with collection of fluid within the obstructed intestine and in the peritoneal cavity owing to transudation, they have usually been vomiting, their plasma flow has been reduced, and their diaphragms are elevated because of distention with subsequent early pneumonia. Then when perforation occurs because of inadequate treatment of the obstructing condition and with it the attendant peritoneal soilage, the mortal blow has been struck.

In general, the sicker and more infirm the patient with intestinal obstruction is, the greater the likelihood for strangulation to occur. Thus, the treatment for such a patient should be more aggressive with earlier laparotomy for relief of the obstruction. Prolonged use of intestinal intubation in such patients should be avoided. Since it is often difficult during the time that a patient with intestinal obstruction is being observed to determine when and if strangulation is occurring, all these patients must be treated with an eye toward the possibility and all concerned must be alerted to this dangerous complication. There is a direct correlation between the length of time that a patient has been obstructed and the probability of strangulation occurring. All bowel that is completely obstructed is subject to the possibility of having its blood supply compromised, with subsequent necrosis.

The patient with intestinal obstruction, regardless of the cause, has abdominal distention, nausea and vomiting, anorexia, crampy pain, hyperperistalsis, and absence of flatus and stool by rectum. Patients with intussusception and volvulus may have a palpable mass either abdominally or by rectal examination; patients with incarcerated hernias may have a palpable mass that is tender. The incidence of strangulation is highest in patients with volvulus and intussusception, and it is also much higher in those with femoral and incisional hernia than it is with inguinal hernias. In the latter case, the rare type of hernia "en bloc," which may falsely appear to be reduced without actually reducing the bowel from the sac, must be considered. Any sudden change in the physical findings and the status of the patient with intestinal obstruction must be evaluated for the possibility of bowel strangulation. A sudden leukocytosis; elevation in fever; increase in tachycardia; fall in blood pressure; rise in the hematocrit, LDH, or SGOT; change in the character of pain from that of crampy to steady, diffuse abdominal pain; shoulder pain; and the disappearance of bowel sounds may herald strangulation with perforation. The development of more rebound tenderness, diffuse spasm, and referred rebound to a specific area must also be sought.

X-ray examination can be of great value in the management of patients with intestinal obstruction before strangulation occurs and as an aid in confirming or diagnosing strangulation obstruction (Chapter Three).

When strangulation has occurred resection is always necessary and a decision about how much bowel to remove must be made at the time of operation. The possibility of leaving some questionably viable bowel and reoperating in 24 to 48 hours in the case of massive strangulation with volvulus of the small intestine may be necessary for survival of the patient.

FOREIGN BODY PERFORATION

Ingestion of any foreign body can be responsible for perforation of the small or large intestine anywhere along its course. Such things as toothpicks, fish bones, and pins have been responsible for perforation. Because there is no apparent reason for the sudden onset of peritonitis, exploration is often delayed. Fortunately, many of these foreign bodies perforate slowly and permit a local walling-off process around the perforating site. There are certain sites at which there is a greater frequency of perforation by such objects (Figure 11–7). Foreign bodies may or may not be visible by x-ray examination. Depending upon whether free or localized perforation has occurred, the appropriate signs will be found by the examiner. The diagnosis can usually be made only at the time of abdominal exploration and even then the cause of the perforation may remain completely unexplained. The offending small foreign body may be within an abscess cavity, be evacuated by the suction, and never be identified. The search for the etiology of the perforating lesion may be frustrating in these cases.

CECAL RUPTURE SECONDARY TO DISTAL COLONIC OBSTRUCTION

There are three major etiologic mechanisms for this tragic occurrence. First, an obstructing carcinoma in the

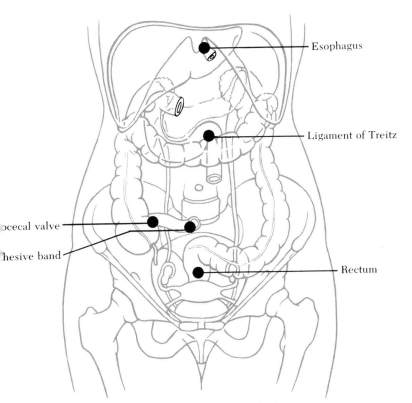

Esophagus

Ligament of Treitz

ocecal valve

hesive band

Rectum

FIGURE 11–7   Sites where an ingested foreign body is apt to perforate or obstruct.

left or sigmoid colon; second, a cecal or sigmoid volvulus; and third, an impaction of the distal colon by either feces or barium often associated with fibrotic or strictured distal colon from underlying disease. Cecal rupture, whatever the etiology, is exceedingly lethal. Cecal contents are very toxic, and an "endotoxin" type of shock will develop soon afterwards with gram-negative septicemia, marked splanchnic bed dilatation, volume deficit, intractable hypotension, high fever, and acute renal failure.

The history is usually one of progressive marked abdominal distention with failure to pass flatus and stool for several days prior to the episode. There is usually a palpable loop of right colon and cecum.

The best way to avoid cecal rupture is to observe carefully the flat film of the abdomen in patients with distended abdomens. If the cecum reaches a size of 12 to 14 cm. by direct measurement, decompression is essential whatever the etiology of the distal obstruction. At a time prior to perforation, prophylactic decompression can be performed either by transverse colostomy or cecostomy, often under local anesthesia. The etiologic basis for the dilatation of the cecum may determine what type of decompressive procedure is chosen. Once cecal rupture occurs, diffuse and rapid soilage of the peritoneal cavity will take place since there is no walling-off of such distended bowel. The patient will rapidly go into shock, with diffuse abdominal rigidity, pain, rebound, tenderness, total loss of bowel sounds, labored respiration, and high fever. The surgical treatment of choice depends upon the etiology of the obstruction. A Mikulicz resection of the perforated segment may be the best procedure in the extremely ill patient.

VASCULAR LESIONS OF THE SMALL BOWEL WITH NECROSIS

All mesenteric vascular lesions eventually proceed to compromise the blood supply with gangrene and perforation of the intestine. Ideally, it is best to avert this by proper relief of the obstructing vascular lesion or adequate resection prior to the time of perforation. Once perforation has occurred, if there is an offending arterial lesion it is still wise to remove the embolus or carry out thrombectomy if this is feasible and then to do an end-to-end anastomosis in viable bowel. Again, it may be necessary to do a limited resection and reoperate in a day or two rather than resect all questionable bowel lest so massive a small bowel resection compromise survival.

Other vascular lesions of the small bowel that can produce perforation and necrosis are periarteritis, fibrinoid degeneration of disseminated lupus, other collagen disorders, and all the usual types of arteritis. Multiple small punctate areas of perforation can occur in such conditions and the extent of bowel to be resected may be deceptive. Vascular abnormalities of the extremities may also affect the intestine, particularly the small intestine. Any of these vascular lesions may rapidly produce full-thickness necrosis of the bowel in the form of a pinlike perforation without any progressive signs. Microscopic study of these lesions reveals the typical arteritis with subsequent full-thickness necrosis. Such patients, when they do have abdominal symptoms, should be observed very carefully with the possibility of exploratory operation held under consideration.

ESOPHAGEAL PERFORATION

Spontaneous perforation of the esophagus may produce signs identical to those of upper abdominal perforation. Such spontaneous perforation usually occurs after a bout of vomiting or retching and produces a typical linear tear just above the cardia, usually above the diaphragm, but it is conceivable that this could be within the abdominal cavity. Air in the mediastinum, pleural effusion, shoulder pain, and dyspnea may be accompanying features. A swallow of methylene blue with aspiration of the left pleural cavity and identification of the dye in the pleural space is the classic way of making this diagnosis. Barium or Gastrografin swallow can reveal the lesion roentgenographically. The history of retching is important, especially when the patient describes inability to produce any gastric contents with this continued vomiting. This tends to rule out an obstructing lesion in the stomach or duodenum and might properly direct the attention of the examiner to the esophagus as a possible source of difficulty. Early repair of the perforation may permit satisfactory recovery before mediastinitis and pneumonia intervene. Time is of the essence just as it is with perforation within the abdominal cavity.

NONPERFORATIVE ACUTE UPPER ABDOMINAL LESIONS

12

ACUTE PANCREATITIS

There are essentially four types of acute pancreatitis that lend themselves to classification: acute edematous pancreatitis, acute hemorrhagic pancreatitis, acute exacerbation of a chronic pancreatitis (chronic relapsing pancreatitis), and acute postoperative pancreatitis.

The acute edematous pancreatitis is the most benign of these four. It often has its onset after a heavy meal or other dietary indiscretion. It frequently is associated with biliary tract disease but not necessarily with common duct stones. Rarely, in patients with familial hyperlipemia an acute crisis of the disease may be associated with pancreatitis.

The onset of pain is usually acute and diffuse, involving the entire epigastrium, with poor localization, and often radiates through to the back. It is a steady type of pain without any crampy component; nausea, vomiting, and often severe retching are associated with it. All the findings of acute upper abdominal peritonitis may be present on physical examination ranging from localized epigastric tenderness with some rebound to severe spasm, rigidity, ileus, and diffuse rebound. In its most severe form, the patient may be in shock from acute plasma volume depletion.

Laboratory aids may be particularly useful in the diagnosis of edematous pancreatitis. The level of serum amylase elevation does not necessarily correlate with the amount of tissue damage or the severity of the disease. It merely quantitates the amount of enzyme in the blood at any given moment. The serum amylase may reach the astronomic proportions of 3000 to 4000 Somogyi units per 100 ml. of serum (normal up to 120 units per 100 ml.) and in those cases is absolutely diagnostic for pancreatitis. Frequently the amylase may only be elevated for the first 24 to 48 hours, and then characteristically the lipase remains elevated for several days. The patient may be jaundiced, since this disease often can be associated with common duct obstruction. The serum calcium may fall as calcium soaps are precipitated owing to the destructive action of the enzymes on fatty tissue. Serum calcium, phosphorus, and alkaline phosphatase determinations should be obtained for all patients with pancreatitis since the possibility of hyperparathyroidism must always be investigated in this disease. Peritoneal or pleural aspiration may be of particular usefulness in making the diagnosis of acute pancreatitis when there are massive elevations of the amylase in the body fluids. Sometimes a distinct advantage, this is not usually necessary for diagnosis. One of the most important observations is the status of the hematocrit, which in this disease reflects the degree of plasma volume deficit, since elevation in the hematocrit is a direct result of the reduction in the circulating plasma volume. This is a much better index of the degree of tissue destruction than the serum amylase level. Pancreatitis associated with hypotension may initiate acute tubular necrosis on the basis of this plasma volume loss into the retroperitoneum; this type of patient has a grave prognosis.

Pulmonary complications occur in 20 to 50 per cent of the patients with acute pancreatitis and may vary from mild atelectasis to fulminating respiratory failure. However, pleural effusions are the most common intrathoracic complications and probably are caused by the transportation of the enzyme-rich fluid through the lymphatics of the diaphragm. The effusions occur more frequently on the left side and subside spontaneously as the pancreatitis improves or can be eliminated by aspiration. These patients need careful respiratory support.

In general, this disease should be treated in a conservative manner, making it critical that the diagnosis be differentiated from one requiring operative intervention in the abdomen. The treatment should be directed toward replacement of any volume deficit, reduction of all stimuli to the pancreas for the relief of pain, and prevention of any secondary peritonitis. Nasogastric suction; careful fluid and electrolyte management; the use of plasma expanders such as plasma, albumin, and blood; antibiotics; antispasmodic therapy; and narcotics such as meperidine (Demerol), which have less effect on the sphincter mechanisms of the pancreatic duct system, should all be employed in the treatment of this disease.

Operative management is indicated in two situations: (1) If the general status of the patient continues to worsen with evidence of biliary obstruction. Under these circumstances decompression of the common duct, usually in the form of a cholecystostomy but occasionally in the form of direct choledochostomy, may relieve the situation. (2) Pseudocyst formation, with or without infection, that is of a progressive nature. Under these circumstances either drainage of the pseudocyst internally, marsupialization of the cyst, or common duct decompression may be indicated. Not all pseudocyst formation associated with acute pancreatitis of the edematous nature need be treated surgically (Figure 9–2). If the diagnosis of acute pancreatitis is uncertain in the patient with an acute abdomen, exploratory laparotomy may be indicated as well, primarily to establish a diagnosis.

Acute hemorrhagic pancreatitis is a much more severe situation than any of the other classes of this disease. It is generally lethal and is thought to have a vascular basis for its development. Necrosis of the pancreas occurs with massive bleeding into the gland and often around it. Severe volume deficit and an elevated hematocrit, prolonged hypotension, and dehydration and associated fever occur. Generally the patient is in severe pain with generalized abdominal signs, particularly with radiation of pain to the back and directly in the midline. The serum amylase is often very low, or often no amylase can be detected in the blood. The main management is massive volume replacement of both blood and plasma to maintain cardiac output and renal function, and the institution of continuous peritoneal lavage. Antibiotics also should be given in high dosage because of the secondary peritonitis that may follow. Surgery may be necessary to debride the necrotic pancreatic tissue and drain any residual pancreatic tissue that is still viable.

This disease is difficult to differentiate from arterial or venous mesenteric vascular occlusion, dissecting aneurysm of the aorta, leaking abdominal aneurysm, and other such major catastrophes. Often the patient has had no previous attacks to indicate that pancreatitis is the offending lesion and, in fact, there is some evidence that previous attacks of pancreatitis may protect patients from this lethal form.

EXACERBATION OF CHRONIC PANCREATITIS

Patients suffering from recurrent pancreatitis usually present as chronically ill individuals who have lost a great deal of weight, have had frequent bouts of recurring epigastric pain, and often have narcotic and alcoholic problems. (All these patients have psychiatric aspects to their disease, which further confuse the physician and the surgeon.) The patient with chronic recurrent pancreatitis commonly has an alcoholic background, but biliary tract disease alone may be the precipitating cause. The pain is usually severe, radiating through to the back and possibly around to the sides, and often there is a palpable tender mass in the epigastrium. The extent of the inflammatory reaction in the pancreas is responsible for the variation in the symptoms. The pain itself is due to obstruction of the pancreatic ductal system, often at multiple sites. X-ray examination of the abdomen usually reveals calcified pancreatitis with fine stippling throughout the whole gland as well as pancreatic lithiasis with stones within the major ductal tree. These patients usually have steatorrhea due to a long-standing destructive fibrotic disease of the pancreas; if no gross steatorrhea is present, high fecal nitrogen levels, much undigested muscle in the stool, and a high fecal fat content are found. Diabetes mellitus develops as there is progressive islet cell destruction along with exocrine loss. Jaundice due to intermittent common duct obstruction and pseudocysts of the pancreas may be associated with chronic pancreatitis. Since these patients suffer from a marked decrease in pancreatic enzymes in the gut, the serum amylase may not be elevated with acute attacks because the gland is incapable of raising the blood level of amylase.

The combination of an epigastric mass, recurring attacks of severe pain radiating to the back, abnormal digestive function, and pancreatic calcification points to chronic relapsing pancreatitis. Jaundice helps to clinch the diagnosis. The possibility of carcinoma in the pancreas can never be completely excluded without a tissue diagnosis, since pancreatitis of this nature can be associated with the development of the tumor. An upper gastrointestinal x-ray series may aid in this diagnosis, particularly when a pseudocyst is present and deforms the stomach or the duodenal loop.

The management of this disease should start with an initial trial of conservative therapy in all cases since this is a chronic recurring problem and a great deal depends on the doctor-patient relationship, the patient's social and dietary habits (particularly if he or she is an alcoholic), and whether or not any surgical therapy is planned. Surgical management should be directed primarily toward providing adequate internal drainage of obstructed pancreatic ducts. The acute pancreatitis that represents an exacerbation of this disease should be treated in the same manner as edematous pancreatitis.

Jaundice may require decompression therapy for treatment. Usually rest without any oral intake will make the symptoms subside rapidly.

Acute postoperative pancreatitis is discussed in Chapter Eighteen.

MESENTERIC VASCULAR OCCLUSION: VENOUS OR ARTERIAL

Both arterial and venous mesenteric vascular occlusion may be insidious in onset; the diagnosis may be obscure, yet the patient may be moribund when first seen. Neither of these situations occurs without some predisposing cause. In the arterial group there may be an embolus from the heart or the aortic wall. Patients with recent myocardial infarctions, ventricular aneurysms, atrial fibrillation, or any type of rheumatic heart disease must always be suspected of having embolic phenomena when they have abdominal pain. A large number of patients also have progressive occlusive disease of the superior mesenteric artery, celiac artery, and inferior mesenteric artery. Often, two of these three vessels are completely occluded, but the collateral circulation from the third is sufficient until progressive occlusion of that vessel occurs; then the entire intestinal vascular tree becomes deficient and massive infarction occurs.

The patients with progressive arterial insufficiency of the intestine may complain of abdominal angina, which consists of diffuse pain after eating. No localized signs are present, but small bowel x-ray may demonstrate distorted bowel function. These patients are particularly vulnerable to "spontaneous" infarction of the intestine associated with low-perfusion states such as myocardial infarction or congestive heart failure. The blood supply is barely adequate for bowel function and viability, and any systemic problem that reduces it further tends to produce infarction of the most susceptible areas—a lesion indistinguishable from superior mesenteric artery occlusion.

Venous occlusion is even more rare. It may occur in patients with volvulus and other congenital malformations and bands. Otherwise it occurs in severely ill patients with chronic congestive heart failure, cirrhosis of the liver, or late malignancy with retroperitoneal involvement and obstruction or partial obstruction of the portal system. Patients with ascending thrombophlebitis or pylephlebitis may present with mesenteric vascular venous occlusion.

Thus, the history and general status of the patient may be extremely important in making the diagnosis. When first seen by the surgeon, patients with mesenteric vascular occlusion are often in deep shock. High fever, leukocytosis, and diffuse abdominal signs accompany evidence of acute plasma volume deficit. Occasionally one may find the patient complaining of severe deep abdominal pain, lying in bed moaning in great distress; yet, aside from mild distention of the abdomen there may be very little in the way of abdominal findings. Rigidity, spasm, localized tenderness, or rebound may be absent. The physical findings generally are determined by the presence or absence of bowel perforation (see Chapter Ten). Aside from distention, the physical examination in the patient who does not have perforation may show decreased peristalsis; diffuse, poorly localized tenderness; and generalized systemic symptoms consistent with acute volume deficit and impending shock, if the latter is not already present. One of the most important findings may be revealed in the pelvic and rectal examination: the presence of blood in the stool. Its absence does not rule out these vascular lesions, since they may be sudden with immediate cessation of peristaltic activity. Frequently a large, boggy, tender, and somewhat movable mass in the pelvis may represent small bowel with compromised blood supply. The presence of ascites may also help in the diagnosis. Nausea and vomiting are often present on a reflex basis. The typical finding on x-ray examination of the abdomen is generalized small bowel distention with some evidence of thickening of the wall and ascites. Since the diseased bowel may not be filled with air, air-fluid levels are frequently absent.

The most important laboratory finding is the elevated hematocrit. Any patient who is moribund, complains of deep abdominal pain, is acutely ill, and has an elevated hematocrit must immediately be considered as having either pancreatitis or mesenteric venous vascular occlusion. Arterial vascular occlusion also can produce an elevation of the hematocrit, since there is trapping of plasma within the infarcted bowel, but the venous occlusion produces a much more significant rise in the hematocrit.

The initial management is replacement of the circulating blood volume. Abdominal exploration cannot be tolerated in the face of shock and inadequate perfusion. Plasma must be given in amounts adequate to replace the deficit as estimated by the changes in the hematocrit. Return of the hematocrit to normal will rapidly follow adequate plasma replacement and this can be used as an index. Vasoconstrictors should be avoided if at all possible. Among the great dangers in patients with hypotension, ischemia, and damaged arterial capillary systems in the gut is the trapping of volume as in endotoxin shock or the occurrence of true endotoxin shock due to bowel damage. Full volume replacement until central venous pressure rises and the use of vasodilators may be indicated as well as appropriate antibiotics.

As soon as the patient can undergo general anesthesia, and this usually can be accomplished in a matter of a few hours of intensive fluid therapy and cardiac management, abdominal exploration should be carried out. Ascitic fluid is always present with devitalized bowel; the usual findings in arterial lesions are either dark, partially necrotic bowel or pale ischemic segments. If the major superior mesenteric artery is occluded, there will be a large segment of the bowel that is infarcted with no pulses in the mesenteric system. If the situation of multiple small peripheral occlusions prevails, then there is very little that can be done surgically except to resect any obviously dead bowel. The question of potential viability is always difficult to answer, and frozen section may help. The possibility of reoperation in 24 to 48 hours may be useful to allow further delineation of bowel that will eventually become nonviable, thus preventing use of inadequate bowel for anastomosis. Bowel suffering from venous occlusion is usually more distended and livid with greater fluid exudate both in the lumen and in the peritoneal cavity than that seen in the arterial lesion. The latter may often show skip areas of ischemic bowel that has slight blood flow when it is pricked with a needle; sometimes it is worth dividing a small vessel on the mesenteric surface of the bowel to see if there is any arterial flow whatsoever. Pressure with a glass slide on the bowel at the time of exploratory operation may help to tell whether or not there is any capillary flow within the wall of the bowel. When the status of the bowel is in doubt, it may be wise to repeat the operation rather than to perform any definitive procedure. This is particularly true in patients who have bowel ischemia in the face of hypotension from other sources. Patients who have undergone trauma to the mesentery may also develop venous occlusion secondary to thrombosis that propagates. In this group of patients a wide resection should be carried out because it is impossible to ascertain the extent of the thrombus at the base of the mesentery and any bowel that is inadequately vascularized will not heal at the anastomosis.

SPLENIC INFARCTION AND SPLENITIS

The acute onset of pain in the left upper quadrant in the abdomen may result from one of these splenic lesions, particularly if it has a diaphragmatic component. Radiation of pain is often to the top of the left shoulder and may be pleuritic in nature with pain on inspiration or coughing; this is particularly true if the infarction is on the superior surface of the spleen.

The importance of diagnosing splenic infarct or splenitis is that, in general, these should not be treated as surgical lesions and must be differentiated from something that does, indeed, require a surgical approach, particularly an acute renal infarct or an acute gastric lesion. The history may often provide the clue, revealing a patient with cardiac disease who has had previous emboli or who has concomitant emboli to other areas of the body. "Splinter" hemorrhages should always be sought in the fingers, skin, or eye grounds; and febrile episodes of bacterial endocarditis are diagnostic. The patient with auricular fibrillation, congenital heart disease, or congestive failure should be suspected. The spleen may be increased in size in splenic infarction, but generally it is not, while enlargement is a feature of splenitis. In seriously ill, febrile patients with chronic congestive heart failure, splenic enlargement may preexist, and it is possible that splenic infarction can be superimposed. Any splenic infarct may be a mycotic type of embolic phenomenon, and splenic abscess may develop from such an infarct. In such a case splenectomy is essential. The pain of splenic infarct may be excruciating and duplicate that of renal colic. Angiography of the celiac and renal arteries may be essential to differentiate the diagnosis.

RENAL INFARCT

Infarction of the kidney takes place against a similar background to that of splenic infarction, that is, in the patient with either auricular fibrillation, recent myocardial infarction, or multiple arteriosclerotic plaques of the aorta to provide a site for emboli to arise from, or in the patient with atrial septal defect who has venous emboli. Intrinsic renal vascular disease with plaque formation can also be responsible for renal infarction on a thrombotic rather than an embolic basis, although this is rarer. Septic emboli can produce perinephric abscess or cortical abscess of the kidney. The pain has a very sudden onset and may be associated, in people with fibrillation, with a change in cardiac rate or resumption or cessation of fibrillation. There may be tenderness in the costoverte-bral angle, and the pain has a greater tendency to radiate to the groin, scrotum, labia, thigh, and lower abdomen than in splenic infarction. It may be more posterior at the outset than the pain of splenic infarction. Generalized signs may occur, such as ileus, vomiting, marked tachy-cardia in the nonfibrillator, hypertension, and fever. It is of prime importance to identify the embolus to a major artery very early because in order to prevent destruction of the kidney or a major infarction of the kidney that may be responsible for hypertension at a later time, it is es-sential to extract the embolus as soon after the injury as possible.

The intravenous pyelogram may be of some help, al-though with a major embolus neither side may function. If intravenous pyelogram does not show function of the affected side, retrograde pyelography must be carried out because ureteral stone disease may be responsible for the same symptom complex. The pain with a renal infarct tends to be more steady and knifelike than the crampy pain of ureteral stone, which is discussed later. Retro-grade or translumbar aortograms may be essential both for establishing the diagnosis and localizing the embolus in planning its management. The degree of symptoms usually is related to how much the kidney is involved in the ischemic process. A total vascular occlusion of the kidney will go on to a completely irreversible lesion with atrophy in a matter of a few hours; thus, there is urgency. The lack of blood in the urine, depending on the location of the embolus, may be deceptive. A more peripheral embolus has a greater tendency to cause hematuria than does a major embolic phenomenon because in the latter case no urine at all is being made.

Surgical treatment should be promptly instituted for a major embolus, with embolectomy being carried out whenever possible. More peripheral emboli should be treated conservatively, and partial nephrectomy may be essential at a later time. The etiologic basis for the embolic phenomena should be treated simultaneously whenever possible.

RENAL CALCULUS

Renal colic is one of the most excruciating types of pain commonly suffered by patients. Crampy and intermittent in nature, it usually begins in the flank and is often associated with nausea, vomiting, and ileus. It radiates obliquely down toward the groin and testicles in the male or the labia in the female (Figure 12–1). The pain may go into the upper thigh, and often is associated with a great desire to void. The presence of hematuria helps to confirm the diagnosis, but if complete obstruction is present hematuria may not occur. Previous attacks may be known, but often the patient, particularly the young patient, presents with a story typical of renal colic without any stone disease in the past.

The presence of renal colic is very common in patients who are severely dehydrated. This is a major problem in the armed forces, particularly during the summer months and in the tropics or in combat when soldiers may be without adequate hydration for several days. The association with abnormal dietary intake seems to produce a high incidence of stones in patients who never before had any renal stones.

The physical examination may be remarkably benign

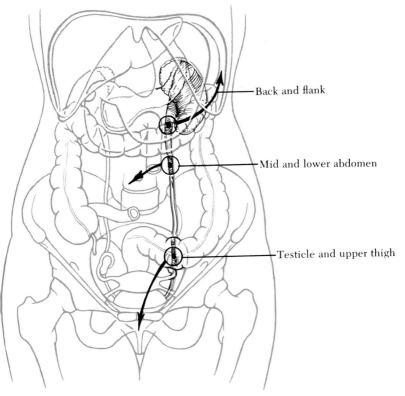

Back and flank

Mid and lower abdomen

Testicle and upper thigh

FIGURE 12–1 Radiation of pain in renal colic.

and this often seems to differentiate renal colic from other acute abdominal conditions. There may be spasm in the flank or along the course of the ureter, and peristalsis generally is reduced.

Intravenous pyelography often may confirm the diagnosis. Even if the obstructing stone cannot be visualized, mild hydroureter and hydronephrosis above the obstructing lesion in the ureter may be the clues. The prevalent sites for obstruction are within the vesical tunnel, at the pelvic brim, and at the ureteral pelvic junction. Occasionally a survey film of the abdomen, if the course of the ureter is accurately outlined, will clearly identify a calcified ureteral or renal stone. It is essential to obtain intravenous urography early before renal shutdown occurs. In all patients with anuria or oliguria, cystoscopy and retrograde pyelography should be performed to rule out the possibility of bilateral obstruction due to stones or to bilateral shutdown associated with colic.

Uric acid levels and multiple serum calcium, phosphate, and alkaline phosphatase determinations must be made in all patients with ureteral colic. Whenever a stone is passed it should be analyzed to arrive at the basic cause for the renal stone disease. Frequently this is never ascertained, but occasionally hyperparathyroidism, gout, or cystinosis may be identified in this manner. Unless marked obstructive phenomena are present in the proximal collecting system, the usual initial management for renal stone disease is directed at giving the stone an opportunity to pass. Operative intervention is reserved for the patient who, despite adequate sedation and hydration, cannot pass the calculus.

CORTICAL ABSCESS OF THE KIDNEY AND PERINEPHRIC ABSCESS

These lesions may be very insidious, and high fever, often unexplained, with a minimum of physical signs may be the only findings. Chills, sweats, weight loss, lethargy, and other constitutional symptoms may be present. Pain may be vague and may be abdominal rather than in the flank. Severe pain may occur with these lesions as well as extreme toxicity. When costovertebral angle tenderness is present it is extremely helpful, but many of these cases do not show this or it may be minimal in nature. Another valuable sign is a change or irregularity in the outline of the kidney by intravenous pyelogram or plain film of the abdomen.

Antibiotic therapy and surgical drainage should be combined in the management of these lesions. The diabetic is particularly prone to develop them and these diagnoses should be thought of more frequently and earlier in patients with diabetes.

RENAL CYST

A simple renal cyst occasionally may produce an acute abdominal problem. Acute hemorrhage may occur into the cyst, or as a result of trauma, rupture of the cyst may take place. When acute hemorrhage is present the onset of pain, swelling, palpable mass, and x-ray changes in the size of the kidney may be noted. Intravenous and retrograde pyelograms may be helpful in the diagnosis, but they usually have to be made on the basis of the physical examination. Fever is rare, but ileus and vomiting may be associated with this type of lesion. Intraperitoneal rupture secondary to trauma will produce a generalized peritonitis and rebound, absence of peristalsis, rigidity, generalized pain, and a shocklike picture, particularly because the bleeding will continue into the peritoneal cavity.

Frequently, a simple cyst need only be partially unroofed and the base, if bleeding, sutured for proper management. It is not essential to resect the cyst unless it easily shells out of the kidney and bleeding cannot be controlled by any other means.

HEPATITIS AND BENIGN HEPATOMEGALY

Conditions such as acute hepatitis, infectious mononucleosis, acute rheumatic fever, or heart failure of an acute nature with hepatomegaly occasionally may cause severe right upper quadrant pain associated with the sudden enlargement of the liver and distention of Glisson's capsule. The pain under these circumstances may simulate an acute abdominal inflammatory process. This is rare, but in seriously ill patients with multiple problems it is possible that this diagnosis can be difficult. The patient with chronic congestive failure or who has had heart surgery for chronic cardiac disease may already have an engorged liver, and then any increase in this engorgement and swelling may produce a change in symptoms that may simulate an acute pulmonary embolus, acute cholecystitis, acute pancreatitis, or a perforated ulcer.

HEPATIC ABSCESS

Hepatic abscess will be considered as coming from four possible sources, its origin being venous (pylephlebitis), hematogenous (via the hepatic artery), or from amebic and echinococcic and other infestations. The general symptoms of hepatic abscess are those of right upper quadrant pain and tenderness, immobilization and elevation of the right diaphragm, and fever that tends to swing with high peaks and troughs in the usual way for abscesses anywhere. The patient may have been chronically ill for several weeks and often has other underlying problems as the basis for development of hepatic abscess. Drenching night sweats, swinging fevers associated with jaundice, and the development of a right upper mass will further confirm the diagnosis. The only basis for suspecting hepatic abscess may be daily, continuous fever in patients who have intraabdominal infection or, in fact, sepsis in any part of the body. Weight loss, lethargy, and anorexia are common constitutional symptoms.

Leukocytosis is usually present when the abscesses are bacterial, but abscesses due to amebic and other infestations involving the liver, especially the tropical type, often are associated with leukopenia and frequently with eosinophilia. Serum chemistry is usually abnormal even if the patient does not have icterus. The SGOT is particularly elevated, as well as the LDH and the BSP levels.

X-rays may be of value since fluoroscopy of the chest will, in many cases, demonstrate elevation of the diaphragm, pleural fluid, and sometimes, in a large abscess, an air-fluid level in the abscess within the liver. Special radiologic techniques, such as the hepatic artery arteriogram or liver scan, may help localize a filling defect within the liver.

Pylephlebitis may occur as a result of intraabdominal sepsis in any portion drained by the portal vein. It is probably still the most common cause of hepatic abscess out of the tropics, except in those situations in which there is direct lymphatic extension from an inflammatory area adjacent to the liver, as with acute cholecystitis.

Acute appendicitis with abscess formation is the classic method for development of pylephlebitis. The infected thrombus eventually may involve the entire portal system, and embolization to the liver may precede direct extension into the liver by the propagating thrombus. In a very grave situation, early diagnosis permits treatment with antibiotics, anticoagulants, and adequate drainage when localization of an abscess can be demonstrated.

The importance of diagnosis of a hepatic abscess must be stressed because of the mortality, which is well over 50 per cent in most series. Posterior abscesses should be drained extraperitoneally through the eleventh or twelfth rib bed; anterior abscesses should be drained from an extraperitoneal approach whenever possible. Embolization to the hepatic artery system, either from hepatic artery aneurysms directly, or from central sources of emboli, including plaques within the aorta itself, may produce a localized infarction of the liver with subsequent necrosis and secondary infection.

Amebic abscess is always secondary to amebic involvement of the colon, but in more than half the cases no active colonic disease is present at the time the abscess is detected. Persistent study of the stool usually produces amebae to confirm the diagnosis. The drenching night sweats, very little icterus, and the general good health of the patient can be compared with the symptoms of one who has a bacterial abscess. Therapy with the proper drug, one of the chloroquine derivatives or the older emetine, often may be diagnostic in demonstrating control of the infection. Surgical drainage need only be contemplated for secondary bacterial infection or failure to control the abscess by drug therapy. The "anchovy paste" color of the mature amebic abscess is classic.

Echinococcic cysts often are calcified; they rarely produce symptoms until they rupture. They may be present in the liver for years and never prove to be a problem for the patient until they either rupture into the free peritoneal cavity, into the biliary system, or into the chest. Biliary tract rupture produces cholangitis and obstruction due to debris; intraperitoneal rupture is very shocking and often is fatal; while transpleural rupture is the least common of the three and may also be very shocking for the patient. Eosinophilia, typical x-ray appearances, skin testing, and complement-fixing studies as well as the proper epidemiologic background may be helpful in the diagnosis.

SUBPHRENIC AND SUBHEPATIC ABSCESSES

Abscesses beneath the diaphragm and around the liver may be very insidious in onset and may occur long after the acute inflammatory process responsible for their inception itself has subsided. They may also occur a few days after perforation of a viscus and may even be present at the time of the initial exploration for a perforated viscus. The diagnosis may be confusing and yet drainage of such an abscess, particularly in the critically ill postoperative patient, may hold the key to survival.

Many attempts have been made to classify abscesses around the liver and the diaphragm according to their location. The liver is attached to the posterior half of the diaphragm in the vicinity of the vena cava and as far medially and laterally as the triangular ligament. Pus can accumulate over the dome of the liver and anterior to the entire surface, in the right lateral gutter, and posteriorly on the border of as well as directly inferior to the liver beneath the gallbladder bed. The entire left diaphragmatic surface is available for collections of purulent material via the foramen of Winslow. The posterior collections of pus are best approached through the bed of the twelfth rib, whereas the anterior ones are best approached by dissecting extraperitoneally until the abscess is palpated. Abscesses on the left side tend to be more deeply seated because they may be protected from the surface by the stomach, spleen, and pancreas, whereas those on the right, because of the very nature of the location of the liver, tend to be nearer the peritoneal surface. Subphrenic abscesses rarely need to be managed as an emergency, and usually it is wiser to be certain of the diagnosis before drainage is attempted.

The diagnosis is similar to that mentioned under the heading of Hepatic Abscesses. The diaphragm above any collection of pus is usually paralyzed, with pleural fluid and atelectasis present above the diaphragm on the side involved. Even paradoxical motion of the diaphragm may be demonstrated by the fluoroscopist. There may be punch tenderness in the involved upper quadrant of the abdomen, abdominal pain on inspiration, pleuritic pain, or shoulder pain referred from under the surface of the diaphragm through the fourth cervical nerve distribution. The most common finding is a spiking, daily fever with a steadily rising pulse rate in a patient who sometimes otherwise feels quite well. Persistent leukocytosis and often positive blood cultures complete the triad. Frequently, antibiotic therapy can avert formation of a frank abscess that requires drainage, but often inadequate antibiotic therapy can make the diagnosis more difficult to arrive at and delay the ultimate drainage required.

When the abscess becomes full-blown, upper abdominal rigidity, tenderness, localized rebound, and pain may be present. Needle aspiration, when successful, is extremely helpful in making the diagnosis, but a negative aspiration, either posteriorly and laterally or anteriorly on the right side, may give the surgeon a false sense of security when it does not return pus. When the diagnosis is considered and it is felt that an exploratory operation is warranted on the basis of the clinical findings, the failure to obtain pus by needle aspiration should not deter the procedure. Frequently such needle aspiration can be done on the operating table with the patient under anesthesia to help the surgeon make the proper approach to the abscess. Whenever possible, extraperitoneal drainage should be carried out, but this may sometimes not be feasible, particularly when the diagnosis is uncertain and a full abdominal exploration is required.

NONPERFORATIVE ACUTE LOWER ABDOMINAL LESIONS

13

PRIMARY PERITONITIS

Under this heading three conditions that present as acute abdominal problems are discussed: bacterial peritonitis (primary), nonbacterial serositis, and mesenteric adenitis.

Primary bacterial peritonitis usually is found in children, since factors of resistance, omental development, and the like seem to play a part in the tendency to develop primary peritonitis. The organism is usually pneumococcus, and the diagnosis can be made with an abdominal aspiration and either a smear or a culture of the fluid obtained. Children with this problem have generalized peritoneal signs without any localization. Pelvic tenderness is also present to a marked degree. There is usually a history of an upper respiratory infection before the onset, but this is not always obtainable. In every case, a localized cause such as appendicitis must be ruled out, and here the disease presents its most difficult aspects. Tuberculous peritonitis at one time posed a similar sort of problem, but was on a much more chronic basis with acute exacerbations. Children with bacterial .peritonitis often have very high fevers, but their general status does not appear deteriorated to a degree commensurate with the fever.

Antibiotic therapy is the treatment of choice once the specific organism is identified; if no identification is possible, treatment for pneumococcal peritonitis should be instituted when the diagnosis is considered. Even when a localized cause of peritonitis cannot be ruled out, while investigation is being carried out and before operation is considered, antibiotic therapy may serve as a therapeutic test to confirm the diagnosis of primary bacterial peritonitis. In adults, although uncommon, some viral infections are capable of producing a serositis or peritonitis. Close observation, frequent examinations of the patient's abdomen, and careful history taking may help to make the diagnosis correctly.

Nonbacterial serositis is a rare disorder that may be on a familial basis. It may be a variant of periodic fever, and often is referred to as familial Mediterranean fever (FMF). The patient presents with signs and symptoms of acute peritonitis with diffuse and severe pain, rigidity, rebound, and cough pain so that at first glance a perforated viscus seems to be the diagnosis. General toxicity is low; pulse rate may often be normal; fever, malaise, and chills are present; and most important, recurrent attacks are the usual history. Often the patient's siblings or parents have had the same problem. It occurs in males more frequently than in females, and usually in people of Mediterranean origin. The great dilemma is that each attack may or may not be a recurrence of a previous situation. It is frequently necessary to explore the patient's abdomen even though the diagnosis is strongly considered. This usually occurs in young people, and an exploratory laparotomy carries very little risk and may help to shed some light on the diagnosis and on the future of that patient. It is important to perform an appendectomy at the time of any operation in such a patient so that acute appendicitis will not have to be considered at each subsequent episode. The peritoneal cavity usually has sterile serous fluid that is clear to opalescent. The entire peritoneal surface shows slight injection without apparent cause.

Mesenteric adenitis is a disease that is also most common in children and young adults. It is usually part of a generalized complex of lymphadenopathy often following an upper respiratory infection. The history of such an infection, of course, is extremely important in making the diagnosis. The pain frequently begins in the right lower quadrant along the chain of the mesenteric lymph nodes (particularly from the ileocecal area), which tend to be the most succulent and enlarged in this disease. The fever tends to be high, 101° to 102° F., with very little evidence of toxicity and not as much localization as is present in appendicitis. The white blood cell count also tends to be higher than in acute appendicitis, at least in its early stage. The onset is often acute; there are very few initial periumbilical complaints and few gastrointestinal tract symptoms such as anorexia or nausea as compared with appendicitis. However, it may be impossible to differentiate this disease from acute appendicitis even depending on fever, white cell count, the remainder of the history, or physical examination. The presence of persistent right lower quadrant point tenderness requires exploration regardless of any other possibilities, and occasionally a patient with mesenteric adenitis will require an exploratory operation. At the time of operation it is often advisable to take a biopsy specimen from one of these enlarged lymph nodes because it is important to differentiate simple mesenteric adenitis from tuberculous enteritis and adenitis, regional enteritis, or lymphoma that may be present in the mesentery. Each of these is discussed later in greater detail. Exploration for mesenteric adenitis when appendicitis is thought to be present results in the rapid subsidence of the abdominal complaint, even though very little is done for the adenitis except to explore the abdomen.

BENIGN INFLAMMATORY GRANULOMAS OF THE SMALL AND LARGE BOWEL

It is rare for benign lesions to present with acute symptoms. Tuberculosis, typhoid, syphilis, and sarcoidosis can all produce ulcerated and granulomatous changes. Occasionally acute perforation occurs. If acute signs develop, operation and local resection are necessary to arrive at the proper diagnosis. The usual findings of pain, local tenderness, and spasm may be accompanied by leukopenia rather than leukocytosis in these circumstances.

LYMPHOMAS AND MALIGNANT LESIONS OF THE SMALL INTESTINE

Most carcinomas and malignant lesions involving the small intestine *per se* usually present as obstructive or perforative problems rather than as acute inflammatory lesions. Occasionally pain of a steady nature without perforation may be the presenting symptom for an inflammatory carcinoma of the small intestine. Frequently a history of some obstruction prior to the onset of this atypical presenting symptom for such a lesion will be revealed by careful questioning. On the other hand, retroperitoneal lymphomas and mesenteric lymphomas may present with acute abdominal pain. Often there is a palpable mass, and there may be other areas of lymphadenopathy to suggest the diagnosis. It may not be possible to make the diagnosis without abdominal exploration in such patients, although lymphangiography, with or without intravenous pyelography and vena cavograms, should make it possible to identify the disease with greater accuracy.

CECAL ULCER

Cecal ulcer may be a solitary, acute inflammatory process, often referred to as phlegmonous, or an acute diverticulitis of a solitary diverticulum of the cecum. Neither of these two could possibly be differentiated except by previous knowledge that a cecal diverticulum is present. Differentiation between these and acute appendicitis or an acute perforation of a carcinoma of the cecum may be virtually impossible. The patient with a cecal ulcer, inflamed diverticulum, or carcinoma may have an inflammatory mass present at the time of the onset of symptoms. Because of the parietal peritoneal location, the onset of pain usually is in the right lower quadrant rather than being periumbilical initially, later radiating to the right lower quadrant as is typical of appendicitis.

INFARCTED APPENDIX EPIPLOICA AND INFARCTED OMENTUM

Both these conditions are quite rare, and it is seldom possible to make the diagnosis prior to exploratory laparotomy. Usually the etiology of their occurrence is never ascertained by the surgeon. They may present with acute onset of pain, frequently in one of the lower quadrants of the abdomen.

PELVIC INFLAMMATORY DISEASE

Pelvic inflammatory disease follows ascending infection in the female genital tract and involves the pelvic portion of the peritoneal cavity (Figure 13–1). Occasionally the main peritoneal cavity can be involved and collections of exudate and adhesions may extend from the pelvic organs to the liver and the diaphragm as a result of previous pelvic inflammatory infection. Although gonococcal infection is the usual cause of pelvic inflammatory disease, it is not always possible to culture this organism at the time of operation or from the cervical os, nor is this the only causative organism. It is most usual for the onset of an acute flare-up of pelvic inflammatory disease to occur just after menstrual flow has ceased, when infection present in the vaginal glands and the cervix ascends through the uterus and out the tubes to involve the pelvic peritoneum.

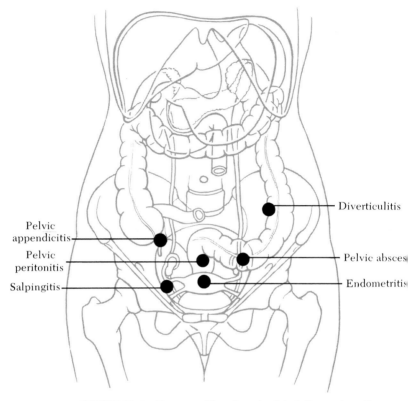

FIGURE 13–1 Causes and location of pelvic inflammatory disease in the female.

The pain is usually lower abdominal and pelvic. The patient complains of a dragging sensation in the pelvis and suprapubic area. It is often steady with radiation to the buttocks, rectum, vagina, and occasionally to the shoulders when any subdiaphragmatic exudation has occurred. With shoulder pain, pain on inspiration may be present and there may be more diffuse signs of generalized peritonitis. These may include evidence of acute plasma volume depletion. Usually the patient complains of a great deal more pain and discomfort than her general appearance would warrant; although the fever may be quite high, she does not appear to be in a very toxic condition with these infections. Lower abdominal tenderness bilaterally usually is found with rebound in the suprapubic area, cough pain referred to the lower quadrants of the abdomen, ileus, and positive psoas and obturator signs. Pelvic and rectal examination is the most specific way to make a diagnosis of acute pelvic inflammatory disease. Without these positive findings on pelvic examination it is virtually impossible to make a clinical diagnosis of acute exacerbation of chronic pelvic inflammatory disease. The presence of discharge from Skene's, and Bartholin's, and the other urethral glands should be checked and appropriate cultures should be taken at the time of examination. Also, material from the cervix should be cultured for any organisms, particularly gonococcus. Usually, the cervix is exquisitely tender on motion in any direction. There may be purulent drainage from the cervix as well. By vaginal and rectovaginal examination, the adnexal areas should be carefully checked for both thickening and tenderness of the tubes and for any evidence of tuboovarian abscesses. It is very common in this disease for an abscess to form between the tube and ovary, particularly because this usually is a recurrent disease and previous adhesions may have formed so that pus can become pocketed between the tube and the ovary, forming a new abscess. By bimanual examination these tender masses usually can be palpated. Frequently no specific masses can be felt but the entire pelvic peritoneum feels boggy and is tender both on bimanual and on rectal examination or vaginal examination alone. Occasionally an abscess can be felt in the pouch of Douglas.

It is infrequent that surgical therapy is necessary as the primary treatment for acute pelvic inflammatory disease. Usually a dramatic response occurs to antibiotic therapy, most commonly penicillin in high doses, as well as to hydration, bed rest, sitz baths, and warm douches. If there is a large tuboovarian mass that is specifically tender it is still wiser to initiate treatment conservatively. If it fails to subside or remains as tender and as enlarged as when first detected, then surgical excision is to be recommended.

The diagnosis of acute appendicitis must be differentiated from acute pelvic inflammatory disease, and it is usually the localization of the pain, the time sequence with regard to the menstrual flow, the physical findings, and the previous history that help to make the diagnosis and separate it from appendicitis. It is important to remember that an acutely inflamed appendix lying on the tube may produce exquisite tenderness when any cervical motion is instituted. At times, differentiation between acute appendicitis and acute pelvic inflammatory disease on a gonococcal or other bacterial basis may be extremely difficult.

FIBROID UTERUS

It is unusual for a fibroid uterus to produce acute abdominal symptoms. It is possible, however, for a pedunculated fibroma, either in the broad ligament or on the free surface of the uterus, to become twisted and to develop infarction with subsequent necrosis. This situation does indeed produce acute pain, frequently poorly localized but generally felt within the pelvis and similar to the pain of pelvic inflammatory disease and menstrual cramps. Occasionally when a fibroid becomes twisted and an infarct develops, there is sudden bleeding within the necrotic tissue and this produces not only pain but pressure and a palpable mass. A further consequence of this acute hemorrhage can be serosal inflammatory reaction with adherence of small intestine and secondary intestinal obstruction.

OVARIAN CYST

No attempt shall be made to classify ovarian cysts here, but any cyst of the ovary can become twisted or cause the entire ovary to twist on its vascular pedicle. Rupture of an ovarian cyst can occur without twisting or it may result from twisting and infarction. It is usually the serous or pseudomucinous cyst that becomes twisted, but certainly a dermoid cyst may become infarcted in this manner. Follicle cysts of the ovary, commonly an aftermath of normal corpus luteum formation, are the type that most frequently rupture and produce local pelvic bleeding with acute abdominal symptoms. Of prime importance in any woman with lower abdominal symptoms is a careful history of the menarche, the time of the previous menstrual period, and the date when the next menstrual period is expected. Follicle cysts usually develop in the last week of the menstrual cycle.

Mittelschmerz, resulting from bleeding occurring at the time of the normal follicle rupture of the ovary, is discussed in another section, but its symptoms and physical findings are no different from those of the small ruptured follicle cyst.

The symptoms from either rupture or infarction of ovarian cysts may be similar to those in acute pelvic inflammatory disease or those described for infarction of the uterine fibroid. The pain tends to be in the pelvis; it may radiate to the vagina or labia, or through to the back. There may be lower abdominal tenderness, and unless the ovarian mass is extremely large it generally cannot be palpated except by bimanual examination. The most common solid type of cyst to become twisted and form an infarct is the fibroma; it is rare for any of the malignant ovarian cysts to become twisted.

One of two situations usually prevails in making the diagnosis. Either the cyst is palpable and exquisitely tender so that the diagnosis of an infarct or at least a twisted cyst is apparent and exploration must be carried out for this reason, or else the patient has persistent lower abdominal tenderness, pain, and spasm and exploration is necessary on that basis rather than because a cyst is palpated. Small paraovarian cysts also may twist and rupture, but this is not at all common.

The twisted or ruptured ovarian cyst, just like the other pelvic inflammatory diseases, may easily be confused with other acute intraperitoneal inflammatory reactions that require surgical care. In most cases they require surgical care for their own management as well as because of the possible presence of some other condition such as appendicitis.

MEDICAL CONDITIONS SIMULATING AN ACUTE SURGICAL ABDOMEN

A number of medical conditions may cause abdominal pain and simulate an acute surgical abdomen (Table 13–1). Acute pneumonic processes, especially those associated with pleuritic irritation, may produce sufficient acute upper abdominal pain, even associated with muscular spasm, to make it important to mention this in the differential diagnosis of the acute abdomen. In addition to fever, cough, and abnormal sputum, the chest x-ray should be diagnostic. A primary pneumonic process must be differentiated from abdominal conditions such as subphrenic abscess, hepatic abscess, and pancreatitis, which may paralyze the diaphragm and simulate a pleural effusion on the x-ray. Pulmonary emboli with infarction on the diaphragmatic surface of the pleura may produce identical findings as well as abdominal pain and spasm. Hemoptysis or peripheral evidence of thrombophlebitis should be searched for and may help to identify the lesions. Spasm and abdominal pain are not associated with other physical findings when pneumonia is their etiology, but sputum examination, including smear and culture, may be critical.

A more obscure disease known to produce abdominal signs similar to those of peritonitis is porphyria. The pain is generally crampy and is frequently out of proportion to the physical findings. Abdominal distention can occur without spasm, and various neurologic

TABLE 13–1 Some Nonsurgical Lesions That May Cause Abdominal Pain

Intraabdominal Diseases:
    Primary bacterial peritonitis
    Salpingitis
    Gonococcal perihepatitis
    Viral hepatitis
    Alcoholic hepatitis
    Mittelschmerz

Extraperitoneal Diseases:
    Pneumonia
    Pericarditis
    Tabes dorsalis
    Porphyria
    Acute pyelonephritis, and cortical renal abscess
    Diabetic acidosis
    Myocardial infarction
    Pulmonary infarction
    Acute pancreatitis
    Periarteritis nodosa
    Polycythemia vera
    Familial Mediterranean fever
    Vascular purpura (Henoch's)
    Chemical (lead, arsenic, thallium, mercury, sodium fluoride, methyl chloride)
    Food (mushrooms, poisoning with staphylococcal and botulinum toxins)
    Retroperitoneal lymphoma

Abdominal Wall Lesions:
    Hemorrhage into rectus abdominus muscle
    Herpes zoster
    Spider bite
    Intercostal neuritis

and psychiatric symptoms may coexist. A history may be elicited of recurrent bouts of similar pain, often precipitated by barbiturate administration. Phosphobilinogen can be identified in the urine of these patients.

An unusual manifestation of diabetes mellitus may be a sterile peritonitis associated with the dehydration of uncompensated diabetic acidosis. The general status of the patient usually leads to the proper diagnosis, and the abdominal pain disappears with hydration. Abdominal crises of tabes dorsalis may be accompanied by severe abdominal pain, like those of paraplegic crises, far out of proportion to the physical findings. Many drug reactions or sensitivities may be associated with diffuse abdominal pain without spasm, and careful history taking and observation are necessary to identify these situations.

Familial Mediterranean fever (FMF) is often a familial disease and is confined largely to those of Jewish extraction. The main feature of the disease is that the patient is well between crises, which strike suddenly with fever, severe abdominal pain, and vomiting. Improvement follows quickly if the patient is given colchicine.

Sickle cell anemia is a hereditary type of hemolytic anemia which is more or less confined to blacks. These patients are liable to crises in which they have sharp abdominal pain. Examination of a moist blood smear shows the sickle-shaped deformity of the red blood cells. After the diagnosis of sickle cell anemia is made, the patient must be observed carefully to decide whether the pain is actually due to a crisis or an acute surgical disease. Patients with sickle cell disease are prone to develop gallstones.

Ascariasis can cause abdominal pain and vomiting and must be kept in mind when the patient lives or comes from a region in which infestation with *Ascaris lumbricoides* is common.

INTESTINAL OBSTRUCTION

SECTION 4

UPPER GASTROINTESTINAL OBSTRUCTION

14

Intestinal obstruction is classified here by the location of the obstruction, starting with the lower esophagus and proceeding to the anus. For ease of description, the symptom complex and the physical signs for obstruction involving certain areas of the gut are grouped together, and then the specific lesions responsible are discussed in more detail. The most common sites of intestinal obstruction are shown in Figure 14–1.

Obstructing lesions are dangerous to the patient in three general ways. First, they produce a catabolic state. The patient is unable to take in adequate nourishment, and until the offending problem is corrected his or her glycogen and fat stores are being broken down to provide calories for normal basal metabolism and additional energy to meet the requirements of the disease state. Second, there is an outpouring and shifting of fluids and electrolytes from the normal compartments into the intes-

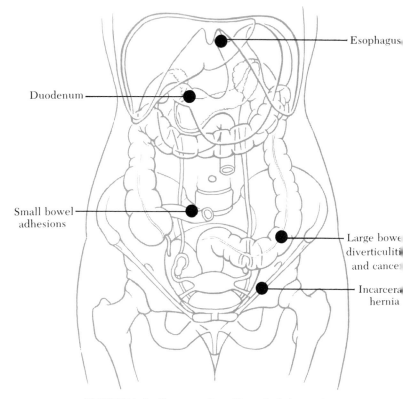

Esophagus

Duodenum

Small bowel
adhesions

Large bowel
diverticulitis
and cancer

Incarcerated
hernia

FIGURE 14–1 Common sites of intestinal obstruction.

tinal lumen and the peritoneal cavity as well as external losses by vomiting and tube drainage. Because rapid changes in both electrolyte and acid-base balance can occur under these circumstances, a careful accounting must be kept of the patient's metabolic balance. Third, and most dangerous to the patient, any obstructing lesion can compromise the blood supply to the proximal bowel with subsequent perforation, adding insult to injury. Prompt diagnosis of the site and probable cause of obstruction and aggressive, well-planned management of the patient with an obstructive lesion of the intestinal tract are essential.

OBSTRUCTION OF THE LOWER ESOPHAGUS

The major symptoms of esophageal obstruction are vomiting, regurgitation, and marked dysphagia with a feeling of food and drink sticking behind the sternum. Vomiting usually occurs shortly after eating, and there is no evidence that any digestion of the food has occurred. Confirmation of the diagnosis depends on esophagoscopy and barium swallow.

The possible offending lesions are: (1) hiatus hernia with reflux esophagitis and stricture formation sufficient to produce obstruction, (2) perforation of the esophagus with mediastinitis and subsequent obstruction, (3) incarcerated hiatus hernia, and (4) carcinoma of the esophagus. Other lesions such as achalasia are not considered here since we are only concerned with acute obstruction.

GASTRIC OBSTRUCTION

Those lesions of the stomach and duodenum that can be responsible for obstruction of the stomach are: (1) chronic duodenal ulcer, often with acute activity; (2) carcinoma of the stomach; (3) acute gastric dilatation following injury or surgery; (4) prolapsing folds of the antrum, a rare cause of gastric obstruction; and (5) prolapsing gastric polyp into the duodenum obstructing the pyloric channel, also a rarity.

Whatever the cause for gastric outlet obstruction, distention of the stomach with vomiting and eructation are the presenting findings. There is usually not much pain within the abdominal cavity, and frequently the gastric dilatation has been progressive so that the patient is hardly aware of it. Dyspnea and shoulder pain may accompany the dilatation. Vomiting may occur long after eating and may be as infrequent as once a day. The patient may notice that the vomitus contains his or her entire oral intake for a period of one, two, or three meals. Marked fluid and electrolyte depletion occurs in patients with obstructing lesions of the stomach, but the degree of electrolyte loss is greatly dependent on the character of the gastric secretion in any specific patient (Chapter Three). The more highly acid the gastric secretion (that is, the lower the pH), the more hydrogen and chloride ions will be lost and the less will be the sodium loss with relatively greater metabolic alkalosis. It is essential, when treating an already depleted patient with an obstructing lesion of the stomach, to analyze an aliquot of gastric juice for sodium, potassium, and chloride concentrations in order to determine the daily requirements for replacement of past and ongoing gastric losses. The character of the vomitus, particularly the presence of bile, is helpful in denoting the level of obstruction since gastric, duodenal, and high jejunal obstructions all present very similar pictures clinically. Benzidine, pH, and volume measurements should be carried out on all samples of vomitus.

Of the five mechanisms for gastric obstruction listed,

only acute gastric dilatation could be construed as being an acute situation producing acute abdominal findings. The others tend to be progressive or repetitive.

Acute gastric dilatation usually can be detected by the plain and upright films of the abdomen in which a large air-fluid level is visualized in the dilated stomach. The patient generally has eructation and vomiting as well as upper abdominal discomfort, and the fluid losses from acute gastric dilatation following surgery or injury can be immense. The best therapy is to empty the stomach with a tube as quickly as possible and to maintain it well decompressed until the underlying etiologic factor is corrected.

During the course of constant suction, careful attention must be paid to fluid and electrolyte replacement. This is true of all obstructing lesions, particularly high obstructions in which there is a disproportion between the various electrolyte ions being removed. Further down in the intestinal tract the electrolyte relationships are more like those in plasma and, therefore, less rapid changes in the acid-base balance result from prolonged suction. Since the proper treatment for acute gastric dilatation is nonoperative, its identification becomes more critical.

DUODENAL OBSTRUCTION

It is extremely difficult to differentiate between duodenal obstruction and gastric obstruction. As with the stomach, many of the conditions responsible are not acute but rather subacute or chronic lesions capable of producing complete obstruction. It must be made clear, however, that in all these situations the patient may not seek medical attention until obstruction has supervened; therefore, he or she may often present to the doctor as a patient with acute high intestinal obstruction, be it duodenal or gastric. A point of differentiation between duodenal and gastric obstruction may be the presence of bile in the vomitus or in the material aspirated from the stomach, although most duodenal obstruction occurs in the proximal portion, so the vomitus would be acholic. Whenever possible, gastrointestinal x-ray studies are most valuable to delineate the diagnosis much more successfully than any other technique.

The various diagnoses that should be considered, aside from an obstructing duodenal ulcer, are (1) carcinoma, either a primary duodenal carcinoma or metastatic carcinoma involving the duodenum intrinsically or extrinsically; (2) superior mesenteric artery compression; (3) annular pancreas; (4) abnormally placed ulcer such as is seen in the Zollinger-Ellison syndrome; (5) malrotation of the gut with an adhesive band to the cecum obstructing the duodenum; (6) intestinal duplication with obstruction as a result of the duplicating loop becoming dilated or inflamed; (7) pancreatitis, particularly of the chronic relapsing type with pseudocyst formation and duodenal compression. The upper gastrointestinal series should be extremely helpful in delineating each of these, at least providing information that helps to differentiate one from the other because of the characteristic types of obstruction produced by each of these lesions.

The presence or absence of jaundice may help to identify the carcinomatous lesion. Primary carcinomas tend to occur in the area of the ampulla, and common duct obstruction might be an early consequence. Carcinoma of the pancreas with invasion of the duodenum is the most common type, and this also tends to produce common duct obstruction with jaundice. Pancreatitis with pseudocyst formation sufficient to produce duodenal obstruction also produces some degree of common duct obstruction in the process.

Patients with superior mesenteric artery compression frequently give a history of pain after eating, usually to a minor degree, and it is rare for this to cause complete obstruction. The non-beta cell islet adenoma or carcinoma producing the Zollinger-Ellison syndrome rarely produces complete obstruction by its size alone, and the accompanying ulcers in various locations in the duodenum have a greater tendency to bleed than to obstruct. The bleeding problem is discussed in Chapter Seventeen.

The patient with malrotation and band formation across the duodenum may never have had any previous history of difficulty and yet can enter the hospital with a complete volvulus of the small bowel rather than simple duodenal obstruction. This may be the most acute of all these situations.

The annular pancreas is uncommon, usually occurring in the second portion of the duodenum and associated with recurrent attacks of obstruction. When complete obstruction of the duodenum ensues, therapy is variable depending on the etiology of the lesion, and no attempt is made to discuss the various therapeutic approaches in this book.

SMALL INTESTINAL OBSTRUCTION

Obstruction of the small intestine may be on either a mechanical or functional basis. The most common type is that due to some actual mechanical obstructing factor that requires a surgical procedure for relief. Many of these lesions are identified in Figure 14–2. On the other hand, functional or physiologic obstruction occurs when the bowel lumen is patent but the bowel is unable, because of its failure to have adequate peristaltic activity,

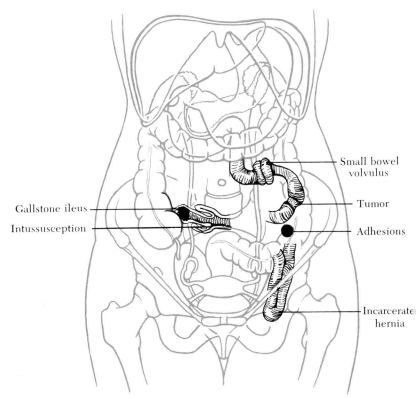

Gallstone ileus

Intussusception

Small bowel volvulus

Tumor

Adhesions

Incarcerate hernia

FIGURE 14–2   Causes of small bowel obstruction.

to propel its contents and it becomes dilated and distended. Occasionally, patients with paralytic ileus, which is common following abdominal surgery, may go on to develop a mechanical obstruction as well, or the ileus may be so protracted and severe that a surgical approach becomes essential for decompression. In general, however, paralytic ileus, when it can be differentiated adequately from mechanical obstruction, does not require surgical management. Thus, as in the patients with acute abdomen due to inflammatory lesions, the important decision in patients with small intestinal obstruction is whether they require surgical intervention. Once this decision is arrived at, surgical intervention should not be delayed any longer than is necessary to prepare the patient adequately for surgery.

The greatest danger in intestinal obstruction is necrosis of bowel caused by prolonged obstruction with secondary vascular changes associated with mechanical obstruction. Bowel may be totally or partially obstructed in a small hernia or other small dependent crevice; as that bowel becomes swollen with its own luminal fluid, edema within its wall increases and its own blood supply may become compromised. Strangulation and perforation are the end results. There is no substitute for swift relief of the mechanical obstruction once it has been decided that a mechanical factor is responsible.

ETIOLOGY

The most frequent cause of mechanical small bowel obstruction is the adhesive band. These bands may be present from the time of birth (congenital) or more frequently are related to some previous surgical trespass within the peritoneal cavity. Bands run either between loops of intestine or from a loop of intestine to the peritoneal wall. Omentum may be involved in adhesions and make a major contribution to the production of bands.

Hernias make up the next most common group responsible for small bowel mechanical obstruction. The majority of these are external hernias. They can be inguinal (direct or indirect), femoral, incisional, umbilical, lumbar, Spigelian, pelvic floor (enterocele), diaphragmatic, or hernia en masse, which is really a type of inguinal canal hernia. None of these become significant with regard to obstruction until small intestine rather than just omental contents and properitoneal fat protrudes into the hernia sac. In the case of the incisional hernia, the base of the sac is narrow and undistensible; these are often associated with incarceration and obstruction. It should not be construed that incarceration in itself indicates obstruction. Nonetheless, a hernia that has been previously reducible and that then becomes incarcerated has a high chance to develop obstruction because something about the hernia and its contents has changed.

Internal hernias are those such as herniation within the ligament of Treitz, which occurs because of faulty formation of the ligament, hernias through pelvic floor repairs, and hernias after other abdominal operations resulting in such things as inadequate closure of a mesenteric rent, tears in the omentum, Roux-en-Y loops that are inadequately tacked down, and ileal loops and ileostomies and colostomies around which the loops of small intestine can become entangled and obstructed.

Whenever any external hernia becomes enlarged, tender, or incarcerated, the possibility of intestinal obstruction should always be raised. Whenever any patient has intestinal obstruction, all sites of possible hernias should be checked at the onset.

Volvulus is a serious cause of small intestinal obstruction because of its high incidence of strangulation. Loops of small intestine of various sizes can become totally twisted within the peritoneal cavity. This differs from the simple adhesive band on which a loop of bowel becomes twisted. This type of volvulus, with only a short segment of bowel involved, is quite different from midgut volvulus. In the latter the small bowel mesentery is abnormally elongated and adherent in its attachments so that is has the opportunity to rotate on itself. Once rotation beyond 180 degrees has occurred the possibility of complete obstruction becomes very high, although 360 degrees' rotation is necessary for this. It then becomes a closed loop obstruction that cannot decompress itself. Rapid progression of symptoms may be the first clue that a volvulus is involved. In addition to adhesive bands, an aberrant or retained vitelline artery, either patent or fused, running from the distal ileum to the umbilicus may induce volvulus of the small intestine. The amount of bowel that gets through the offending bandlike structure of the internal hernia or the amount that is twisted in the midgut volvulus is critical to the outcome for the patient, when and if strangulation occurs. In most of the adhesive band situations only a small amount of bowel is involved and, although strangulation is more frequent, the ultimate survival of the patient is not endangered as long as resection is performed early enough. Midgut volvulus, which is often associated with a transverse band across the duodenum and a misplaced cecum with cecal volvulus, tends to involve the entire small bowel, and if infarction does occur, the lesion is incompatible with life.

Intussusception is most common in children, but also may occur in adults if some leading point (intussuscipiens) is present to initiate the process. Ileoileal, ileocecal, and colocolic are the three most likely types of intussusception in the adult. Intussusception is often associated with a palpable mass and blood in the stool and also deformity of the abdomen with an unsymmetrical appearance on physical examination.

Tumors of the small intestine, both benign and malignant, must be considered as causes for intestinal obstruction and often are the leading points for intussusception. Polyps, fibromas, leiomyomas, lipomas, and adenomas (other than mucosal polyps) are examples of the benign lesions, while leiomyosarcomas, carcinomas, and lymphomas are the type of primary malignant lesions encountered. Carcinoids also may cause obstruction, although they are usually so slow growing that this is unusual. Metastatic carcinomas more commonly cause obstruction than primary tumors, often at multiple sites in the small intestine.

Endometriosis can produce small bowel obstruction both by the extrinsic pressure of inflammatory cysts and by the cyclical inflammatory reaction causing plication-like kinking of bowel, one loop against the other. The cyclic nature of the history is the key to the diagnosis.

There are a host of chronic granulomatous lesions such as regional enteritis, tuberculosis, sarcoidosis, and syphilis that are capable of producing acute small bowel obstruction, although often another chronic illness with recurrent obstruction is also present. However, it is not unusual for an acute attack of regional enteritis to present as small bowel obstruction in its initial episode. This is much less common with typhoid, tuberculosis, and lues.

Abscess formation as a result of perforation of other organs, as in acute appendicitis, tuboovarian abscess, colonic diverticulitis, and peptic ulcer disease, makes use of loops of small intestine to wall-off the septic process and localize the abscess. Once this is accomplished, the loop of small bowel may become edematous, inflamed, and obstructed.

Ileostomy dysfunction is a type of small bowel obstruction that may be very severe and disabling to the patient. Since, in a sense, an ileostomy is a surgically created fistula, there is constantly an attempt on the part of the skin of the abdominal wall to constrict and close it. If improper healing has occurred or trauma is present at the mucocutaneous junction, narrowing of the lumen will occur. The most common site for this narrowing is the mucocutaneous junction rather than the muscular layers of the abdomen. Ileostomy dysfunction associated with partial obstruction, rather than decreasing the amount of efflux, usually is associated with ileostomy diarrhea, since hyperactivity of the ileostomy and of the proximal ileum occurs to surmount the partially obstructed site. Tremendous quantities of intestinal juices and their associated electrolytes may be lost in a matter of a few hours, and hypotension with potassium depletion with its associated cardiac difficulties can ensue.

Congenital duplication of the small intestine producing a loop of bowel with a common wall to a functioning loop of intestine may produce obstruction in rare instances by becoming dilated and impinging on the lumen of the functional loop.

Gallstone ileus is also a rare occurrence that takes

place when a large gallstone in the patient with chronic cholecystitis erodes through the gallbladder into the duodenum. The gallstone then is carried along into the small intestine until it reaches a point where it cannot pass. The common sites are the ileocecal valve, the ligament of Treitz, or any previous adhesion. Of course, stones pass down the common duct and into the duodenum, but these are never large enough to produce obstruction of the small intestine such as occurs when a large stone erodes through the gallbladder directly. The finding of air in the biliary tree on a flat film of the abdomen is an important key to the diagnosis of gallstone ileus because the offending stone may not itself be visualized.

Pain is the most prominent and reliable symptom in a patient with mechanical small bowel obstruction. The pain usually is generalized and primarily central in the periumbilical area and is of a crampy, intermittent character. Nausea, vomiting, and anorexia usually are associated with the pains, but do not necessarily coincide in a synchronous manner with a rush of abdominal pain. The nausea and vomiting are generally of a reflex nature in the initial phase, but as progressive distention of the stomach and reverse peristalsis occur, these produce vomiting. Usually, the patient has not passed any flatus or had any bowel movement for several hours, but patients with high obstruction may continue to have bowel movements for about 24 hours as the bowel has a chance to empty itself. As the period of obstruction continues, the vomiting, which initially may have been clear and bile-stained, becomes feculent because of the static bacterial growth within the distended bowel over this long period of time. The signs of systemic toxicity are not a part of small bowel obstruction, but as the fluid and electrolyte loss becomes severe, as the bowel becomes more edematous, and as bacterial toxic products become absorbed, these signs appear. It may not be possible to differentiate the toxicity of prolonged small bowel obstruction from that of superimposed strangulated bowel, and at that stage rapid intervention and relief from the obstruction become urgent.

SIGNS

Abdominal distention is the most basic finding owing to dilatation of the proximal loops of bowel with gas and fluid. Occasionally, loops of bowel may actually be palpable in a thin individual, and the hyperperistaltic activity can be seen by just looking at the abdominal wall and watching the waves of muscular contraction moving along these dilated loops. Some diffuse abdominal tenderness may be present, but at the onset there is very little tenderness, just distention, and the distention may not be marked initially. The degree of vomiting or suction that has been applied to the upper gastrointestinal tract helps to determine the degree of distention present. The need to check all possible sites of hernias as an initial part of the abdominal examination in anyone who is obstructed cannot be stressed too often, since an incarcerated, tender hernia may be the immediate tip-off to the diagnosis. Auscultative examination reveals rushes of peristalsis with high-pitched sounds and these correlate identically with the pains that the patient complains of. This is a most important point in differentiating mechanical obstruction from paralytic ileus. The patient with paralytic ileus can never show this degree of hyperactivity, since by definition the smooth muscle of the small intestine is incapable of it.

The hematocrit coupled with the daily weight is useful for following the general hydration status of the patient, especially when one is trying to maintain a rough intake and output balance for extrarenal losses of fluid and electrolytes. A rise in the hematocrit always indicates plasma volume deficit due to inadequate volume replacement under these circumstances. A fall in the hematocrit may be less certain, but can represent overhydration or chronic blood loss. The white blood cell count may be extremely important since the white cell count and differential count should be relatively normal at the onset of a simple small bowel obstruction, but if any damage to bowel develops, as toxicity increases the white cell count begins to rise. The level of serum amylase may be moderately elevated, perhaps twice normal, in the face of obstruction alone because of the more efficient reabsorption of these enzymes from the damaged mucosa of the obstructed gut. This is usually still below the level that would be diagnostic of primary, acute pancreatitis. The lactic dehydrogenase (LDH) level is generally of not much help until necrosis of bowel occurs; then it may be very significant, as would be the SGOT. Blood urea nitrogen and the serum electrolytes should be observed because they are all indications of fluid and electrolyte balance as well as of renal function. In high jejunal obstruction or obstruction of the duodenum the bilirubin and alkaline phosphatase may also be important. Benzidine-positive stool may indicate neoplasm or strangulation of the involved bowel. Of all the laboratory aids, the x-ray examination generally proves to be the most valuable both in making the diagnosis and in following the patient pre- and postoperatively (Chapter Three). The use of barium or other contrast medium by mouth should be limited to small amounts of a soluble opaque medium, through a Miller-Abbott tube if possible. The disadvantages of a regular barium meal to locate a small or large bowel obstruction are, first, the barium fills the entire bowel so that further radiologic examination of the abdomen is worthless; second, the large amount of barium remains in the intestine postoperatively and may contribute to impaction problems; and third, the bolus of barium might convert a partial obstruction into complete obstruction. Information may be obtained by instilling a small amount of dye and then getting sequential films to see where the obstructing site is. Sometimes it is very difficult to differentiate clinically between the paralytic type of ileus and a mechanical obstruction in such patients, and the persistence of the opaque medium at a certain point over a period of several hours helps to identify a specific lesion.

TREATMENT

One of the major problems with intestinal obstruction, in addition to the danger of strangulation, is the abnormality in fluids, electrolytes, and acid-base balance that occurs when large amounts of gastrointestinal fluids are aspirated or vomited. Ileostomy dysfunction often starts with diarrhea, as mentioned, and a massive potassium loss can occur in a short time. These patients tend to be potassium depleted to begin with, and under these conditions metabolic alkalosis quickly ensues and cannot be corrected until the postassium loss is corrected. It is important to have a concept of what the electrolyte losses are from the stomach, the upper small intestine, the lower small intestine, and the colon in patients with intestinal obstruction, so that some clinical grounds can be established for replacement of ensuing and prior losses. Table 2–3 provides the ranges of electrolyte concentrations in common body fluids.

Some general points about the treatment of mechanical obstruction are mentioned, but no attempt is made here to go into any detailed surgical review. The treatment consists, first of all, of making the diagnosis and differentiating it from paralytic ileus. It is not always possible to make the specific diagnosis of the etiology of obstruction, but in general, mechanical obstruction requires surgery, and, once diagnosed, surgery should be planned. The patient who is in good condition and has been obstructed for only a short time does not need much delay for fluid replacement. On the other hand, the severely debilitated, elderly, or toxic patient will tolerate operation and the postoperative period much better if you at least begin fluid, electrolyte, and acid-base repair prior to and during the operative procedure rather than trying to pick up the pieces, so to speak, after mechanical obstruction has been relieved by surgery. Patients who are alkalotic and hypokalemic will be made worse by anesthesia and surgery *per se* even if the obstruction is relieved. Initiation of repair should be carried out whenever possible prior to the actual operative procedure. Generally, the more critical the patient's condition, the sooner the operative procedure should be performed, since these patients can afford the least mismanagement. Everything must be done just right for them to survive the episodes of obstruction, and the sooner this episode is relieved the better off they will be.

When the operation is performed for intestinal obstruction it is imperative for the surgeon not only to relieve what appears to be the cause of obstruction, but to examine the entire small intestine and large intestine carefully to be certain that the only cause of obstruction has been relieved. Other adhesions should be removed, especially those distal to the point of obstruction, and a careful search should be made for small bowel tumors at the same time. Sometimes partial obstruction, due to a more distal lesion, can initiate a full-blown mechanical obstruction due to an otherwise innocuous adhesion in a more proximal locus, and the surgeon may be deceived into believing that relief of this obvious obstructing site will suffice, whereas in actuality the offender is still present more distally. Complete obstruction proximally allows collapse of the small bowel even proximal to a partially obstructing lesion more distally. Tube jejunostomy performed under light, general anesthesia or under local anesthesia in extremely ill patients may be lifesaving and may permit adequate decompression in a hurry so that the greatly dilated abdomen with elevated diaphragm in a severely hypoxic patient may be alleviated temporarily and permit subsequent full-scale exploratory laparotomy.

LARGE BOWEL OBSTRUCTION

15

Common sites of large bowel obstruction are shown in Figure 15–1. Large intestinal obstruction is frequently of a closed loop type when the ileocecal valve is competent. If this is the case, the cecum may distend rapidly in a transverse or left-sided obstruction and the danger of cecal rupture is great. Vomiting and nausea may occur on a reflex basis. On the other hand, if the ileocecal valve is not competent, then large bowel obstruction produces a picture of small bowel obstruction as well. It may be impossible to distinguish by initial evaluation whether the small bowel obstruction is primary or secondary to a left-sided lesion of the colon. Colonic carcinoma is so common, as is volvulus of the sigmoid in some parts of the world, that the value of a barium enema in patients with low small bowel obstruction as well as large bowel obstruction cannot be overemphasized. It can be performed gently and safely and may often provide the important diagnostic information. Procrastination with large bowel obstruction is dangerous because of the possibility of a

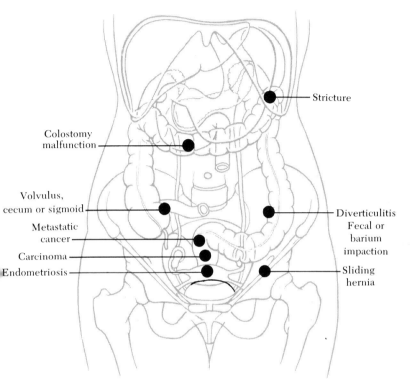

FIGURE 15–1 Causes of large bowel obstruction.

closed loop and the fact that the blood supply to the large intestine is much less adequate than that to the small intestine. Lesions that produce strangulation *per se* are much less common in the large intestine, and the danger is usually of cecal rupture rather than of unidentified strangulation, except with volvulus. The cecum can be evaluated carefully by plain films of the abdomen, and if of a size of approximately 13 cm. in diameter, decompression must be carried out immediately by cecostomy. Once the diagnosis of large bowel obstruction is established a right transverse colostomy is indicated, since the vast majority of large bowel obstructions are due to lesions in the left or sigmoid colon. Occasionally, an obstructing lesion of the sigmoid can be exteriorized and resected.

COLOSTOMY DYSFUNCTION

This diagnosis is generally fairly obvious. Stricture of colostomy is usually at the site of the cutaneous anastomosis, much as in an ileostomy. It is unusual for the muscular portion of the colostomy to become obstructed in an adult. The patient may have noted difficulty inserting the catheter if he irrigates his colostomy, or narrowing of the stool from the passage through the colostomy. Patients are very aware of their colostomies, and the diagnosis is usually not difficult. Colostomy dysfunction is associated with distention, crampy pain, and constipation, and obstipation may go on to a full-blown picture of obstruction. Revision of the colostomy in such instances is mandatory.

FECAL AND BARIUM IMPACTION

This presents a similar picture to colostomy dysfunction, except that the entire bowel is in place. Constipation of a chronic nature is a very common complaint, particularly in the elderly in whom bowel activity is even more sluggish. Cathartics usually are resorted to, and these produce chronic potassium depletion, which in itself tends to make the bowel function even worse. It is possible for an elderly person confined to bed for several weeks, particularly with a chronic injury such as a fracture, to develop a chronic fecal impaction in the colon. Frequently, diarrhea is associated with this at first as an attempt is made to bypass the impaction by maintaining a liquid stool, but eventually the entire rectum and sigmoid may be completely occluded with inspissated feces.

This is not always seen only in the elderly since adolescent girls, particularly when they have emotional problems, tend to be constipated and can have large impactions that produce distention, cramps, and abdominal masses. Patients who have chronic constipation may develop barium impaction following incompletely evacuated barium enemas, and these become even more inspissated than stool alone because the barium content becomes hardened.

Most of these can be relieved by digital disimpaction; the diagnosis usually can be arrived at by the presence of stool throughout the large intestine without any specific point of narrowing.

CARCINOMA OF THE COLON

Carcinoma of the right side of the colon rarely produces obstruction because the lesion, although large, is slowly growing in an area of the bowel that tends to be more distensible and where the stool is more liquid. Carcinoma of the right side of the bowel usually produces anemia due to chronic bleeding, with a palpable mass and weight loss completing the triad of presenting findings. Occasionally, carcinoma at the hepatic flexure may produce obstruction with rapid distention of the cecum and usually secondary small bowel obstruction. It is particularly difficult in these patients to palpate the carcinoma at the time of exploratory laparotomy; the surgeon often needs the assistance of the barium enema to identify the obstruction site. As the location of the lesion progresses toward the splenic flexure and the left side of the colon, obstruction occurs at a relatively earlier time in the life history of the tumor. It takes about 12 to 18 months, it is estimated, for a tumor to become circumferential in the bowel and usually obstruction does not occur until the tumor resembles a napkin ring almost entirely surrounding the bowel.

In general, the patient who enters with obstruction due to a left-sided carcinoma has been having low-grade bowel symptoms for 2 to 3 months; occasional crampy pain, narrowing of the stool, and difficulty in moving the bowels that requires more straining. Sometimes some bleeding has been associated with this, but this is not necessarily a gross finding by the patient. Sigmoidoscopy is extremely important since 75 per cent of the lesions of the large intestine are within view of the sigmoidoscope. Fifty per cent are within reach of the palpating finger, but the lesions that obstruct are usually in the sigmoid, the narrowest part of the bowel being the intraperitoneal sigmoid. These are generally above the level of the examining finger, so that for obstructive lesions the sigmoidoscope is usually important. On the other hand, bleeding lesions are often within the rectum; these are usually palpable by the examining finger. Along with cramps and dilatation of the abdominal wall, patients with obstructing lesions often complain of tenesmus and diarrhea.

If sigmoidoscopy can demonstrate the lesion it is usually unwise to perform a barium enema at this stage. Barium might get through the lesion; the fluoroscopist, because of the distention and fecal material present, would not be able to ascertain whether or not a proximal lesion is present; and the barium would only add to the impaction. If the sigmoidoscopic examination does not reveal an obstructing lesion and evidence of large bowel obstruction is present, then a barium enema should be performed very gently to identify the exact site of the lesion.

A right transverse colostomy is performed to decompress the left colonic obstruction and at a later date the primary lesion is resected. The transverse colostomy is closed subsequently, completing the three-stage operation. The alternative method of treatment is primary resection plus a temporary proximal colostomy, a two-stage operation.

DIVERTICULITIS

Diverticulitis frequently produces obstruction of the left colon in the area of the sigmoid. It can coexist with and may be difficult to differentiate from carcinoma, although the finding of an inflammatory process may help. Diverticulitis often produces a tender mass right at the pelvic brim, which is palpable by both abdominal and rectal examination, with a febrile response, whereas obstructing carcinomas may not be associated with any fever. The patient may have a long history of diverticulitis and possibly will have had a previous diagnosis by barium enema.

Sigmoidoscopy should be carried out in all these cases to rule out carcinoma. However, failure to obtain a positive diagnosis of carcinoma when an inflammatory narrowing prevents passage of the sigmoidoscope through the obstructed site does not rule out malignancy. During the time taken for conservative management, diagnostic techniques such as sigmoidoscopy, gentle barium enema, and possibly stool cytology can be carried out. If the obstruction subsides this generally rules out the possibility of obstructing carcinoma, since subsidence, even when an inflammatory element is superimposed, is unusual in obstructing carcinoma. Obstruction due to sigmoid diverticulitis can be relieved by exteriorization of the involved colon or by a right transverse colostomy, and later resection. A primary resection should rarely be performed for obstruction resulting from inflammatory bowel disease; if such a resection is carried out, it must be complemented by a diverting right transverse colostomy.

ENDOMETRIOSIS

Just as it can produce small bowel obstruction, endometriosis can cause large bowel obstruction, particularly on the left, because of extraluminal fibrosis, scarring, and inflammatory cysts. This is not a common lesion, but it should be considered in the female who has premenstrual and menstrual pain, who is in the mid to late portion of her menstrual life, who has had no children, and who has a story of cyclic crampy pain with recurrent attacks of abdominal distention. It is rare for endometriosis to produce complete large bowel obstruction, but this is a possibility since the cysts can enlarge and grow into the bowel mucosa. It is difficult to make the diagnosis prior to operation. Primary resection of the involved colon usually is feasible.

VOLVULUS OF THE LARGE INTESTINE

There are two types of volvulus: that of the cecum and that of the sigmoid. Cecal volvulus is much less common, it comes on very acutely, often with no previous attacks, and massive distention can occur in a short time. The patient is acutely ill with vomiting, massive distention, and crampy pain with dehydration occurring rather rapidly. This is a closed loop type of obstruction at its onset. The loop itself is usually not very long but becomes massively distended and occupies the left upper quadrant. A malrotation or abnormal mobility of the cecum is essential to permit cecal volvulus to develop. The diagnosis can be suggested on x-ray by the massively distended cecum misplaced out of the right lower quadrant into the left upper quadrant (Figure 3–10). Operative procedure should consist of reduction of the volvulus and fixation of the cecum in the right lower quadrant; right colectomy is essential if there is evidence of strangulation.

Sigmoid volvulus is much more frequent, in places where vegetarian diets are more common, particularly in South America, Iran, and Africa. Sigmoid volvulus occurs much more easily in two situations; chronic constipation and the presence of a long mesentery to the sigmoid.

Hyperperistalsis or constipation encourages recurrent twisting at this preselected point, and eventually a 360 degree or greater rotation occurs producing complete obstruction of a closed loop type. Strangulation may occur very rapidly, but not as quickly as with cecal volvulus.

The major complaints are massive distention, pain, cramps, and obstipation. On x-ray examination there is the typical appearance of the twisted sigmoid coming down to a narrow point in the left lower quadrant where the volvulus begins (Figure 3–9). This corresponds to the point of the twist of the volvulus.

In many instances sigmoid volvulus can be reduced sufficiently by sigmoidoscopy to prevent the need for emergency surgery. Through the sigmoidoscope the twisted site, usually about 15 cm. from the anus, can be identified, and a well-lubricated soft rubber catheter or the sigmoidoscope can usually be inserted beyond the edematous area. Likewise, passage of barium by the fluoroscopist may reduce the volvulus. Either of these should certainly be tried prior to operation. Perforation can occur with these attempts at reduction; this possibility should always be remembered. Even though the bowel can be reduced, the possibility of prior strangulation must not be overlooked. The presence of tachycardia, elevated white cell count, fever, generalized pain, and peritoneal signs may indicate infarction of bowel. Once a volvulus has caused complete obstruction the rate of recurrence is high, and even though it can be reduced permanent therapy still may be required. A short resection of the sigmoid, including the scarred area which predisposes to recurrent sigmoid volvulus, is the best means of repair.

COLONIC OBSTRUCTION DUE TO METASTATIC CARCINOMA

The area of the peritoneal reflection in the pouch of Douglas is the most common site for metastatic carcinoma to produce colonic obstruction, both because of the frequency with which metastases seed there and because the stool is firmest at this location. Ovarian, gastric, cervical, breast, and recurrent colonic cancer are the tumors that most often cause this. Frequently the diagnosis can be arrived at by digital rectal examination or by sigmoidoscopy, this being the classic "rectal shelf." Ureteral obstruction may accompany it and the prognosis is grave. Despite the obviously far-advanced state of the metastatic malignancy, the symptoms can be of rather acute onset. A simple bypass procedure is the treatment of choice when the intraperitoneal site of obstruction is above the pelvic floor; an end sigmoid colostomy may be required for obstruction in the vicinity of the pelvic floor.

HEMORRHAGE AS A CAUSE OF THE ACUTE ABDOMEN

SECTION 5

CAUSES OF ABDOMINAL HEMORRHAGE

16

Patients can present with acute abdominal bleeding either within the lumen of the gastrointestinal tract or freely into the peritoneal cavity. Each of these groups presents distinctly different findings, and different types of management are essential. Generally, those with intraperitoneal bleeding present in shock with an acute peritoneal reaction, whereas those whose bleeding is intraluminal may be bleeding on a more chronic or intermittent basis although massive blood loss and shock are common.

INTRAPERITONEAL HEMORRHAGE

Many of the situations responsible for intraperitoneal hemorrhage are related to trauma. These are discussed in Chapters Eight and Nine. The great bulk of other causes of significant symptomatic intraperitoneal bleeding is either lesions of the vascular tree or related to gynecologic and obstetric conditions in the female (Figure 16–1).

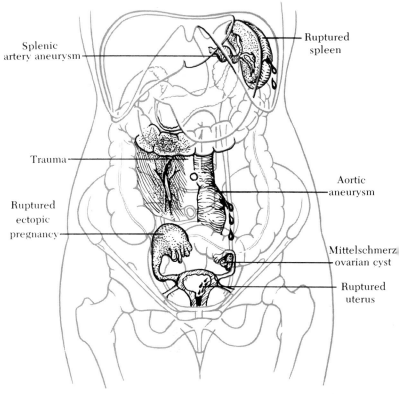

FIGURE 16–1 Causes of extraluminal abdominal hemorrhage.

NONTRAUMATIC SPLENIC RUPTURE

Any massively enlarged spleen such as that present in leukemia, myeloid metaplasia, Hodgkin's disease, malaria, tuberculosis, kala-azar, syphilis, and infectious mononucleosis can rupture as a result of minimal and usually unrecognizable trauma. Also, subcapsular rupture can have taken place with trauma and then, at a time distant from the initial injury, free splenic rupture into the intraperitoneal cavity can ensue. The development of hypotension associated with left upper quadrant pain, abdominal rigidity, and the findings of peritoneal irritation, as well as left shoulder pain, inspiratory pain on the left side, and an enlarged spleen on both physical and x-ray examination, help to support this diagnosis. Abdominal aspiration will support the diagnosis if blood is obtained in the aspirate. As in any other splenic rupture, splenectomy must be done.

RUPTURE OF HEPATIC OR SPLENIC ARTERY ANEURYSM

These are both rare lesions, but bleeding from either of them can be massive and fatal in a very short time if not properly treated. A previous flat film of the abdomen may be extremely useful in arriving at the diagnosis, since both these aneurysms tend to have a rim of calcification that can be identified on the x-ray. It is possible that either may leak slightly before massive rupture, so that the presence of posterior abdominal pain with peritoneal findings may be sufficient evidence to make the diagnosis by either of two methods. The first of these is the palpation of a thrill on examining the upper abdomen, in splenic artery aneurysm just to the left of the midline, in hepatic artery aneurysm to the right of the midline. Second, by auscultation a murmur may be heard that is usually loud, systolic, and transmitted over a fairly

large area in the upper abdomen. The aneurysmal sac
may not be more than a centimeter or so in diameter, but
the diagnosis of rupture can be entertained, although it is
of little import in the management of the patient. With
either of these aneurysms bleeding, the patient enters the
hospital with hypovolemic shock. After blood volume has
been replenished with massive transfusions, an exploratory operation should be performed with great haste.
There is little time to attempt diagnostic evaluation by arteriography; the diagnosis usually will be arrived at on
the operating table when the site of bleeding is identified. Hepatic artery aneurysms are usually in the main
hepatic artery, making resection difficult.

The splenic artery aneurysm presents no difficulty,
since the artery can be ligated proximal to it and splenectomy carried out. Occasionally, other aneurysms in the
celiac axis are associated with it, particularly those of
the left gastric artery along the wall of the stomach, and
these should always be looked for in such cases. Aneurysms such as these can be oversewn at their site and
nothing further done about them. Frequently aneurysm
of the splenic artery occurs right at the hilum of the spleen
and leads to a mistaken diagnosis of spontaneous rupture
or traumatic rupture of the spleen. It may be necessary to
employ a thoracoabdominal approach to remove the massively enlarged spleen.

ABDOMINAL AORTIC ANEURYSM

Three types of problem with the abdominal aneurysm will be mentioned. First, the dissecting aneurysm
that arises in the ascending aorta. It may dissect around
the renal arteries, the celiac, the superior or inferior

mesenteric and, in fact, down each iliac artery. It is possible that somewhere within the peritoneal cavity it will rupture through the adventitia, producing massive intraabdominal bleeding. If this is the case it is rare that the patient even arrives at the hospital prior to death. On the other hand, the dissecting aneurysm may have come on acutely and may not have dissected either through the adventitia or back into the lumen, and the patient may present with severe knifelike back pain, hypotension, radiation of pain down the back to the legs or to the flanks. If the dissection has occurred into the wall of the aorta without rupture in either direction, pulses in the groin may be decreased but still present. The patient at that stage may not be in a state of shock; this is the ideal type of patient to be salvaged by intrathoracic repair of the dissection. The diagnosis must be differentiated from acute myocardial infarction, massive pulmonary embolus, or a ruptured or dissecting standard abdominal aneurysm. The latter will be discussed later. These first two diagnoses have multiple other modes of differentiation: the electrocardiogram, the history, and blood studies. If the patient has the characteristics of Marfan's syndrome with the webbed neck, finger abnormalities, and a family history of similar episodes, this may lend credence to the possible diagnosis. Widening of the mediastinum on the chest x-ray should also be seen, since the origin of aortic dissection is in the ascending arch. Whether time for retrograde aortography is available depends on the individual case; if it is, the diagnosis can be arrived at more definitely by this technique. Any catastrophic abdominal pain with or without hypotension should always have dissecting aneurysm and enlarging or bleeding abdominal aneurysm in its differential diagnosis.

Abdominal aortic aneurysm can be a stable situation, in which case it is usually completely asymptomatic and presents with a pulsatile, palpable mass or if lined with clot may be identified only by the plain film of the abdomen. The lateral film of the abdomen particularly demonstrates the eggshell calcification of the anterior surface of the aneurysm that permits its diagnosis. This type of aneurysm will not be the subject of discussion here. On the other hand, the general rule is that if these aneurysms exceed 6 cm. in diameter they will tend to bleed at some time, usually within 2 years of the time the diagnosis is arrived at. The knowledge of such an aneurysm should be carefully impressed on any patient so that if he or she has the onset of acute abdominal pain, its presence will be realized.

A leaking aneurysm either may rupture anteriorly—providing free blood in the peritoneal cavity, rapid collapse, hypotension, and anuria—or it may rupture posteriorly—in which case there will be massive distention and retroperitoneal bleeding but the inflammatory reaction around the back of the aneurysm will maintain the patient's viability for a longer time and permit him or her to get to a hospital with a greater chance for survival. The survival rate from bleeding aneurysms, however, is only 10 to 15 per cent in most series. Excruciating, steady back pain, often with absence of pulses in the lower extremities, hypotension, and distention, rapid shock, anxiety, and sweatiness indicate the diagnosis. This may be confirmed by palpating the pulsatile abdominal mass, usually tender when bleeding occurs. As soon as the patient is seen, cutdowns should be placed, massive transfusions should be begun, and he or she should be taken to the operating room as quickly as possible. Once the abdomen is opened, pressure should be applied to the aorta above the aneurysm to get control of the bleeding and maintain flow to the heart and brain. This is the only approach for survival of the patient because cardiac arrest may rapidly follow the induction of anesthesia.

ACUTE ABDOMINAL FINDINGS ASSOCIATED WITH NORMAL MENSTRUAL VARIANCE

MITTELSCHMERZ. As its name implies, mittelschmerz is pain in the middle of the menstrual cycle. It is common and frequently occurs month after month or in the majority of the months in a woman's cycle. Often, therefore, the woman is well aware that the pain that may occur acutely is that of mittelschmerz. This is pain associated with rupture of the follicle and passage of the ovum through the wall of the ovary. It is probably due to bleeding that produces a local peritoneal reaction in the vicinity of the ovary. Since either ovary can produce active graafian follicles, the pain can occur on either side. When it occurs on the left it presents little problem, but the right lower quadrant pain must always be differentiated from acute appendicitis.

On occasion, the pain of follicle rupture may be severe indeed and may necessitate abdominal exploration. This may occur even in the face of previous attacks of mittelschmerz that were not nearly as painful. The character of the pain may often be similar enough so that the patient can identify it; if this is the case, despite the severity of the pain, careful observation may lead one to the right diagnosis since it is a self-limiting problem.

Naturally, the most important factor in the diagnosis is a history of the menstrual cycle, with this pain coming on anywhere between 10 and 20 days after the previous period or 14 days before the next expected period. The pain is often acute at onset and frequently in the right lower quadrant rather than radiating from the periumbilical area. This is because the irritation is directly to the parietal peritoneum and, therefore, immediate localization occurs associated with the onset of pain.

REFLUX OF MENSTRUAL FLOW. A rarer situation is reflux of the menstrual flow out the tube, producing a local collection of blood in the peritoneum near the fimbriated end. This produces physical findings and a history identical to that of mittelschmerz except for the timing. It comes on during the menstrual flow rather than halfway between periods. The possibility of this being acute pelvic inflammatory disease or endometriosis with an acutely distended cyst must also be considered. It is during the menstrual cycle that endometriosis and pelvic inflammatory disease both flare, as does mittelschmerz. If the physical findings are severe and progressive enough to indicate it, exploration should be carried out.

FOLLICLE CYST OF THE OVARY WITH BLEEDING. This problem may be difficult to differentiate from acute appendicitis when it occurs in the right lower quadrant. Follicle cysts of the ovary may be only a centimeter or so in size and represent a small collection of fluid at the site of a follicle into which bleeding may occur prior to rupture. Normally, as the follicle site heals there is minimal reaction. However, if a cyst develops it may rupture at any time. Frequently, this occurs near the time of a menstrual period because of the time sequence required to develop a follicle cyst and for it to rupture.

Only if the follicle cyst is palpably enlarged on rectal and vaginal examination can any clue to the diagnosis be arrived at. Pain is usually present on motion of the cervix, but this is not necessarily so since the irritation is due to the bleeding on the peritoneal surface rather than in the ovary itself. Hematocolpotomy is more likely to be positive for this condition than for menstrual reflux or mittelschmerz, since the bleeding tends to be much more significant from a ruptured follicle cyst. If the cul-de-sac feels at all full and distended, colpotomy certainly should be carried out.

ENDOMETRIOSIS

Generally, endometriosis does not present as an acute abdominal problem. The patient frequently has a story of infertility and of having rather severe menstrual pain. The physical examination may reveal retroversion of the uterus, much thickening and fixation of the uterosacral ligaments, and possibly a mass in one of the ovaries.

Endometriosis can produce acute abdominal situations when a chocolate cyst of either of the ovaries ruptures, producing acute pelvic bleeding, or when a chocolate cyst anywhere else in the pelvic area ruptures to produce acute bleeding.

Acute pelvic bleeding plus the presence of an ovarian mass necessitates immediate abdominal exploration, whether the diagnosis preoperatively is endometriosis with bleeding or a ruptured ectopic pregnancy. In this situation, colpotomy or abdominal tap in the lower quadrant may be of great aid in arriving at the diagnosis. The operative treatment is excision of the abnormal cyst with preservation of ovarian tissue if possible.

ECTOPIC PREGNANCY

In the childbearing age group, a ruptured ectopic pregnancy represents a life-endangering lesion on every occasion. Probably only those ectopic pregnancies in which the test for pregnancy, measuring chorionomogonadotrophins, is positive are capable of producing massive life-threatening hemorrhage. This is because in cases with negative pregnancy tests the placenta is not invasive and the fetus is no longer viable. In such cases the vascular supply to the placenta is usually greatly reduced. Ectopic pregnancy most commonly makes itself apparent 2 to 4 weeks after a period has been missed, which places it at about 1 month of gestation. Many times such an ectopic pregnancy is lost and passes as a missed period, and nothing further comes of it. If it is substantially implanted in the tube, on the surface of the ovary, or even intraabdominally away from the ovary and the tube (i.e., in the back of the uterus or on the sigmoid), such an ectopic pregnancy may indeed produce massive hemorrhage.

There are four significant points in making the diagnosis. The first is that of a missed menstrual period or a markedly abnormal previous menstrual period. Second is the onset of pain in the abdomen, most commonly due to intraabdominal bleeding. The third is intraabdominal bleeding with evidence of volume depletion, tachycardia, hypotension, sweating, and thirst. The abdomen may be distended and have a doughy consistency on examination. Occasionally, vaginal spotting may be present, but this is not necessarily a consistent finding. The vaginal spotting may be due to bleeding down the tube if there is a ruptured ectopic pregnancy in the tube, to changes in the decidual lining of the uterus, or to shunting of the blood present within the uterus at the time of rupture of the placenta and its vessels. The final point in the diagnosis is the finding of a mass on pelvic examination. This mass is not usually very large but may be the clue as to the presence of an ectopically placed fetus and placenta.

Rapid diagnosis and prompt operation to control the site of bleeding are essential. As in any other acute bleeding problem, immediately upon control of the bleeding site the patient's vital signs become stabilized. It is essential that blood replacement be given while preparing such a patient for operation; frequently such massive hemorrhage has occurred that the patient is in deep shock upon arrival at the hospital. Abdominal tap may help to make the diagnosis when a less significant amount of bleeding has occurred. The same is true of colpotomy. If ectopic pregnancy is suspected and the pregnancy test is negative, it is possible to maintain careful observation rather than to immediately explore the patient's abdomen.

INTRALUMINAL GASTROINTESTINAL HEMORRHAGE

17

Anywhere in the course of the gastrointestinal tract bleeding can occur to a degree that requires immediate operative intervention. Many of the bleeding problems in the gastrointestinal tract are of a chronic nature; most have the capability of producing a massive hemorrhage. The most important function of the surgeon and the physician, working together as a team in caring for patients with gastrointestinal bleeding, is to first locate the site of the bleeding and then to treat it. The site of the bleeding is of significance because the chance of massive and life-endangering hemorrhage varies according to the etiologic basis for the bleeding. Bleeding can be divided, particularly, into that from the upper and lower gastrointestinal tract. The ability to obtain blood or guaiac-positive material by aspiration of the stomach with a nasogastric tube may be critical in differentiating one of these from the other. As a result of reverse peristalsis due to the irritability caused by blood in the small intestine, any lesion from the ileocecal valve upward is capable of producing blood in the stomach, although lesions below the ligament of Trietz rarely do this.

Bleeding lesions of the large intestine, especially on the right side, may be easily confused with lesions of the small intestine or even the duodenum, depending on the rate of bleeding and the character of the bloody stool. The history of previous attacks, the age and sex of the patient, other concomitant conditions, drugs the patient may be taking, the presence or absence of vomiting with the bleeding episode, the history of previous surgery, and the results of previous radiologic examinations are points to be investigated in taking the patient's history. As distinguished from other lesions of the acute abdomen, the physical examination in patients with gastrointestinal bleeding may be completely normal. A mass should always be sought in the upper abdomen and the right colon, but aside from these and some tenderness when an acute duodenal ulcer is the cause of bleeding or when acute diverticulitis is present, few other positive physical findings may be noted. It should be pointed out that some of these lesions also can produce other findings and an acute surgical abdomen; that is, obstruction, perforation, peritonitis, and acute inflammatory conditions can always be associated with bleeding from the lumen of the bowel.

Upper gastrointestinal tract bleeding (Figure 17–1) is most commonly due to peptic ulcer, usually duodenal but frequently gastric. To be included with this is the marginal or jejunal ulcer following gastrojejunostomy. Acute gastritis, either of the hypertrophic or atrophic type, may be responsible for massive bleeding; eso-

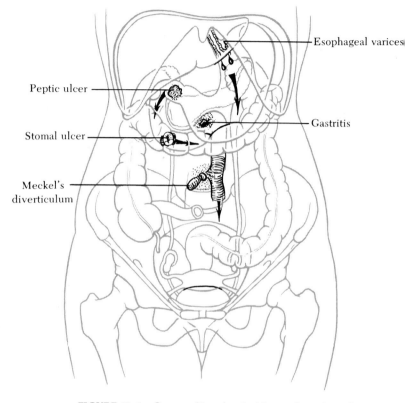

FIGURE 17–1 Causes of intraluminal hemorrhage from the upper gastrointestinal tract.

phageal varices, particularly when the stigmata of liver disease are present, must be ruled out in massive hematemesis. In the elderly patient, often without any previous symptoms, with a slow weight loss and mild obstruction, carcinoma of the stomach must be considered as a cause of massive bleeding. Acute ulceration in a hiatus hernia or associated with incarceration of a hiatus hernia as well as accompanying peptic esophagitis can all bleed. Other types of esophagitis may also produce bleeding, although that associated with hiatus hernia is the most common. Acute bleeding from gastric and duodenal polyps is rare, and even more unusual is the presence of duodenal and jejunal diverticula that can bleed and cause reflux into the stomach. The small intestine can be the site of massive bleeding from lesions such as primary jejunal ulcer, Meckel's diverticulum, regional enteritis, small bowel tumors (benign and malignant), and intussusception.

The diagnosis often may be arrived at by upper gastrointestinal x-ray. The use of the gastroscope, particularly one utilizing fiber optics, has increased the accuracy of such studies. The ability to perform esophagoscopy in a patient in whom varices are under consideration may be important. If time permits, a Miller-Abbot tube or a fluorescine string may be passed to determine the exact site of bleeding in the small intestine. However, determination of the exact site of large or small intestinal bleeding may be uncertain even at the time of laparotomy; under these circumstances multiple enterotomy or colotomy incisions may be required to find the bleeding point.

Bleeding in the large intestine (Figure 17–2) can be more correctly diagnosed by the combination of barium enema and sigmoidoscopy. The fiberoptic colonoscope provides an excellent method to examine the colon and diagnose the cause and site of colonic bleeding. In the elderly, massive bleeding from diverticulosis is certainly a possibility and very difficult to manage since, even at

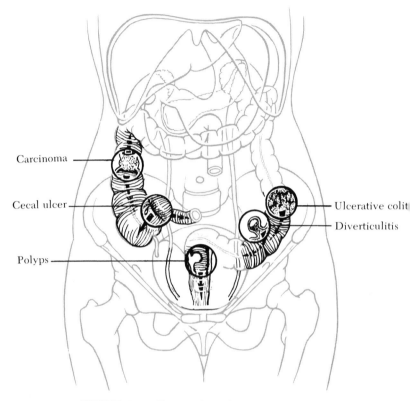

Carcinoma

Cecal ulcer

Polyps

Ulcerative colit

Diverticulitis

FIGURE 17–2 Causes of intraluminal hemorrhage from the colon and rectum.

operation, it is impossible to know just which of the diverticulae may be bleeding. Carcinoma of the large bowel may produce massive bleeding, but it usually ceases without emergency colostomy being required. Diverticulitis bleeds in about 10 per cent of the cases, which makes it even more difficult to differentiate from carcinoma. Ulcerative colitis may produce massive large bowel hemorrhage as its initial finding, but usually it is associated with a previous history of ulcerative colitis. Bleeding pseudomembranous enterocolitis is more diffuse, rarely is life-endangering, and may be associated with pure cultures of *Staphylococcus* on smear in extremely ill individuals. It certainly should be considered in all cases of patients who demonstrate bleeding into the stool with distention, diffuse pain, fever, and long-term illness, particularly if they are on antibiotic therapy. Ischemic colitis or the "ischemic bowel syndrome" occurs in older patients and the left colon seems to be the most vulnerable to the disease. The exact cause of the condition is not known. The main symptoms are mild abdominal pain and the passage of bright red blood by rectum. The mucosal surface of the involved bowel shows edema, a dusky color, and areas of ulceration from the sloughing of the mucosa. Barium roentgenographic examination may show "thumb printing," the most common finding. Colonoscopy can be helpful in the diagnosis since the lesion is usually above the reach of the ordinary sigmoidoscope. Surgical resection is required only if massive bleeding occurs or for late complications such as perforation due to bowel necrosis or stricture formation. Exteriorization of the bowel is the treatment if the bowel is necrotic. Bleeding to a severe degree can occur from hemorrhoids, particularly internal hemorrhoids, and from fissures in the anus to a much lesser degree. On occasion internal hemorrhoids can become very eroded and produce significant spasm so that a great deal of bleeding can occur into the rectum and its ampulla before being noticed on the surface. The large fungating carcinoma of the rectum can produce significant bleeding associated with tenesmus; usually it is easily palpable by finger or visible through the sigmoidoscope, and biopsy specimens can be obtained in this manner.

The lesions of the upper gastrointestinal tract most likely to produce bleeding massive enough to be fatal are those from peptic ulcers, severe acute gastritis, and esophageal varices. A rare cause of massive small intestinal bleeding is the erosion of a pseudoaneurysm of the aorta into the fourth portion of the duodenum. This results from a chronic leakage at the anastomosis of an aortic bypass graft. Ulcerative colitis, diverticulosis, and occasionally diverticulitis in the lower intestinal tract may produce exsanguinating hemorrhages. Bleeding from carcinoma of any portion of the gastrointestinal tract rarely is brisk enough to fit into that category.

It is vital in the surgical control of gastrointestinal bleeding to find the bleeding point, but it is not always easy to do so.

Massive hemorrhage from esophageal varices frequently is treated initially by balloon tamponade with the Sengstaken-Blakemore triple lumen double balloon. Gastroesophageal hypothermia is another medical method of treatment. Specific surgical treatment of a definitive nature is emergency portocaval shunt.

Subtotal gastrectomy is the treatment of choice in massive bleeding from a gastric ulcer, although occasionally excision of the ulcer combined with vagotomy will suffice. There are several alternate surgical approaches to treatment of an actively bleeding duodenal ulcer. Excision of the ulcer with pyloroplasty and vagotomy; subtotal gastrectomy with vagotomy; and simple suture of the ulcer are the methods generally used. The former two techniques are preferable to the latter, which is more applicable when one is treating an elderly, extremely ill patient with multiple system disease.

If the site of bleeding originates in the small intestine, which is not a common location of massive hemorrhage, the treatment is resection and end to end anastomosis. It must be remembered that some tumors of the small bowel tend to be multiple, so the entire small bowel should be examined carefully for other lesions even though the bleeding point has been found.

The surgical management of massive bleeding from the large intestine may be difficult because the exact site of bleeding may be obscure, especially in extensive diverticulosis. The availability of the colonoscope promises to make the examination of the colon more exact in such instances. If the hemorrhage is from the right colon a right colectomy is indicated. Bleeding lesions in the transverse, left, and sigmoid colon are resected with anastomosis with or without a temporary proximal colostomy. Fortunately, under most circumstances bleeding from diverticulosis ceases spontaneously. Occasionally a "blind resection" of a portion of the colon is necessary in which active and persistent bleeding is associated with widespread diverticulosis.

The instillation of vasoconstrictor drugs into the site of bleeding by selective angiography has not lived up to expectations, except in the case of bleeding gastritis. Occasionally active bleeding from colonic diverticulosis is controlled by a barium enema. It is best not to temporize with lesser means in the face of active massive bleeding from the gastrointestinal tract if the bleeding point can be localized and surgically controlled.

THE POSTOPERATIVE ABDOMEN

SECTION 6

THE ACUTE POSTOPERATIVE ABDOMEN

18

The complications of abdominal surgery are legion; some are minor, but many are catastrophic. None is more important than an acute abdominal disease arising and superimposed on a patient who has had a recent intraabdominal operation. The term "acute postoperative abdomen" may include complications directly related to the operative procedure, such as a hemorrhage, or an independent lesion such as acute cholecystitis following a routine hysterectomy.

THE APPROACH

One must have an organized approach toward what may be the cause of the superimposed postoperative abdominal problem. First, the incision itself; infection, bleeding, and dehiscence are obvious complications. Second, what was done? Is a leak from an anastomotic suture line causing peritonitis, or was a nearby organ such as the pancreas or spleen traumatized during the operation? Third, postoperative hemorrhage may occur after any intraabdominal operation. Immediate recognition and treatment are imperative. Fourth, intestinal obstruction can be a serious sequela of major abdominal surgery. Fifth, urinary retention is common after abdominal surgery, but injury to the ureters must be kept in mind. Sixth, injury to large vessels may be the cause of concealed hematomas if not of open hemorrhage. Seventh, unrecognized trauma by instruments such as retractors may be the cause of bleeding from such organs as the liver or spleen. Eighth, metabolic disorders such as previously undiagnosed Addison's disease or diabetes mellitus may become manifest in the immediate postoperative period.

THE UNCOMPLICATED POSTOPERATIVE ABDOMEN

A well-performed major abdominal operation is followed by amazingly little reaction. *Pain* should be minimal and clearly related to the incision. Straining, moving, and coughing will aggravate incisional pain but should be controlled easily by moderate doses of morphine or similar drugs. The pulse rate should be below 100 per minute provided blood loss has been replaced and there are no cardiopulmonary complications. *Fever* is not a reliable sign in the first 48 hours after operation. However, a steadily rising temperature is characteristic of a progressing infection. The liberal use of antibiotics has made fever a fairly undependable sign, since the temperature may be normal or only slightly elevated in the presence of serious infection. The respiratory rate usually is slightly elevated because of incisional pain. Quiet, easy respirations are almost as reassuring as a normal pulse. Rapid respiration in the absence of pulmonary complications is an alarming sign. Acute gastric dilation may be the cause of rapid respirations when other abdominal findings are minimal. Insertion of a nasogastric tube will quickly clarify the cause.

Examination of the abdomen may show mild distention for two days after operation. Auscultation will reveal a few peristaltic sounds during this period; after that they should be readily heard. Palpation, gently performed, away from the incision should elicit no rigidity or tenderness. Percussion may be helpful in identifying a dilated stomach or distended bowel.

DANGER SIGNALS

The danger signals after intraabdominal surgery are persistent pain, tachycardia, rapid respirations, persistent absence of peristalsis, progressive distention, and fever. The experienced clinician usually can recognize at once that the patient is not doing well, and is alerted to find out and correct what is wrong. While this discussion is focused on the acute abdominal problem, the cardiopulmonary system must also be evaluated, the status of the central nervous system determined, and the renal function known. In other words, in the face of the acute postoperative abdomen, the patient as a whole must be assessed even more carefully than before the operation.

THE INCISION

Incisional complications such as bleeding or cellulitis may appear immediately. The diagnosis and the treatment are obvious in these circumstances. The bleeding must be controlled and if there is a cellulitis of the incision the skin sutures should be removed, the wound cultured, and appropriate antibiotics given. If the bleeding is from the skin, sutures can be placed at the site of bleeding under local anesthesia. However, if the hemorrhage is in the deeper layers of the incision, the incision must be reopened and the bleeding point ligated. Merely packing the incision open for hemostasis is to be avoided.

The delayed complications such as abscess, hematoma, and dehiscence become apparent later in the postoperative period (5 to 14 days). These problems rarely are confused with intraabdominal lesions, although ileus or even some degree of small bowel obstruction may be associated with wound dehiscence. Thin, pink, watery fluid exuding from an abdominal incision is characteristic of dehiscence and appears before the entire incision is disrupted. The incision should be resutured at once, either in layers, or with through and through retention sutures, or a combination of both. With an extremely ill person temporary adhesive strapping and a Scultetus binder can be used.

Wound abscesses must be widely drained. This can usually be done without anesthesia by carefully inserting a hemostat gently but firmly through the incision into the abscess cavity. Fortunately, most wound abscesses do not extend beyond the subcutaneous layer. Wound hematomas, if large, should be evacuated; not infrequently they are combined with abscess formation, the so-called "infected hematoma."

ANASTOMOTIC LEAKS

Fortunately, leaks from gastrointestinal anastomotic suture lines are not common, but if not recognized when they occur, may be fatal. Leaks from sutured bowel or stomach may occur any time within 10 days of operation, but are unusual before 48 hours after operation. The first signs of leakage from the gastrointestinal tract are those of peritonitis. They may, however, be masked by antibiotics and sedation. A rising, bounding pulse; a quiet, distended, tender abdomen; and some elevation of temperature are the warning signals. Copious drainage from the nasogastric tube accompanies this picture. The stage of toxemia and collapse may develop before the usual signs of peritonitis are unequivocally present. The search for free air by roentgenographic examination is not too helpful because of the free air that is always present for several days after any laparotomy. Pneumoscrotum may be an early sign of anastomatic leakage of the anterior resection of the rectosigmoid and may appear before the patient shows systemic signs of the leakage. The four quadrant abdominal tap, however, often will make the diagnosis immediately. When the leak is diagnosed, drainage or exteriorization of the leaking area is usually safer than an extensive operation to repair it in a very toxic patient. Sump tube suction drainage is an excellent method to drain the leakage from a disruption of the duodenal suture line after subtotal gastrectomy. With free soilage from a colonic anastomosis an immediate proximal diverting colostomy is mandatory, plus adequate drainage of the site of leakage.

POSTOPERATIVE HEMORRHAGE

This catastrophe usually becomes apparent while the patient is still in the recovery room. He or she shows signs of blood loss despite replacement that was considered adequate for the operative procedure. The rising pulse, lowered blood pressure, diminished urine output, and general appearance of the patient usually make the diagnosis obvious. The best policy is to reoperate on the patient and control the bleeding as soon as the surgeon is certain that the hemorrhage is not caused by uncorrected deficiencies in bleeding and clotting mechanisms. Giving multiple transfusions in the hope that the massive bleeding will stop is inviting failure to save the patient. There are, of course, instances when the bleeding is not rapid or life-endangering in which replacement in volume and careful observation are justified. The surgeon, however, must always ask the question, "Will waiting stop hemorrhage?"

BLEEDING FROM GASTROINTESTINAL SUTURE LINES

Postoperative hemorrhage from a gastrointestinal suture line is more apt to occur after gastrojejunal anastomosis than elsewhere in the gastrointestinal tract. The diagnosis is suggested by the continual passage of blood through the nasogastric tube or by rectum with accompanying tachycardia and hypotension. Once the diagnosis is made, the anastomosis should be exposed and the bleeding vessel ligated. When possible, it is safer to make a separate incision in the bowel either above or below the suture line to identify the bleeding point and ligate it rather than to take the anastomosis apart. When hemorrhage occurs at an anastomosis involving the left colon or sigmoid colon it may be wiser to exteriorize the bowel temporarily, in order to control the bleeding.

INJURY TO ORGANS UNRELATED TO THE PRIMARY LESION

No matter how gently or carefully an abdominal operation has been performed, injury to other structures is possible. For example, the tear in the spleen or liver from a strongly held retractor may cause subsequent bleeding from the structure. A retractor pinching a loop of small bowel may result in pressure necrosis and a late open leak from the bowel. A deeply placed retention suture may perforate intestine and cause a fistula or even peritonitis. Injuries to the urinary bladder and ureters are so notorious they hardly need to be mentioned. Too vigorous exploration of areas away from the incision may tear adherent structures and cause bleeding or flare-up of chronic diseases such as cholecystitis and diverticulitis. These are merely examples of what every surgeon must think of in the patient who develops a postoperative acute abdomen.

PARALYTIC ILEUS

This type of small bowel obstruction is on a physiologic basis. There may be multiple areas of reverse peristalsis and "puddling," but primarily the intrinsic nerve supply to the bowel appears to be interfered with in some way. It is most commonly observed in the immediate postoperative period; after intraperitoneal complications such as peritonitis, perforation, or abscess formation; or with retroperitoneal injury such as spine fracture, retroperitoneal bleeding, and pancreatitis.

After complicated abdominal surgery in which continued peritoneal irritation is present, such postoperative ileus may persist for many days. Under these circumstances there is continued potassium depletion due to upper intestinal suction, and this in itself, unless adequately replaced, may tend to prolong the inadequate muscular tone of the bowel. If ileus of the paralytic nature persists more than 7 to 10 days it becomes increasingly difficult to differentiate it from superimposed early postoperative mechanical obstruction. In fact, the term "ileus obstruction" refers to the situation of prolonged ileus that assumes the characteristics of mechanical obstruction and may require surgical drainage to reestablish the muscle tone of the bowel wall.

An absence of hyperactive sounds in the presence of generalized distention, or a silent abdomen with an occasional distant high-pitched tinkle are the usual auscultatory findings in paralytic ileus. There is usually painless distention, there may be some stool in the rectal ampulla, and vomiting may be present owing to gastric distention. A flat film of the abdomen generally reveals a diffuse pattern with small and large bowel dilatation without any localization or solitary enlarged loops. Perforation of the bowel rarely occurs in paralytic ileus.

INTESTINAL OBSTRUCTION

Mechanical intestinal obstruction, usually of the small bowel, can occur after any abdominal operation. In its early stages postoperatively it is seldom recognized because of the prevalence of paralytic ileus. It may be due to immediate postoperative adhesions, a malfunctioning anastomotic stoma, unrecognized disease such as multiple adhesions distal to the point of a repaired obstructing adhesion, prolapse of bowel into operatively produced defects (i.e., through the new pelvic floor after an abdominoperineal resection of the rectum), or abscess formation. In any event, except in the rare mesenteric vascular complications, the surgeon has some time before a decision must be made to reoperate. In general, paralytic ileus should subside or improve after the first 3 postoperative days, and then it is up to the surgeon to determine whether true mechanical obstruction exists. The diagnosis is not easy, and in this situation intestinal intubation and close observation of the patient are justified.

Radiopaque material instilled via the nasogastric tube or taken by mouth, its course followed by serial roentgenograms, may be necessary to distinguish between paralytic ileus and mechanical small bowel obstruction.

ACUTE GASTRIC DILATATION

Acute gastric dilatation is a distressing and potentially serious complication of abdominal surgical operations. The probable series of events is that the stomach's intrinsic propulsive power is inhibited and swallowed air and gastric secretions accumulate. Gastric distention stimulates further gastric secretion, a vicious cycle. The patient complains of upper abdominal fullness, may hiccough and have nausea and vomiting. Tympany is present over the gastric area and an upright roentgenogram will confirm the diagnosis. However, that is seldom necessary if a nasogastric tube is passed into the stomach; the gush of air and drainage of retained gastric secretions via the tube will establish the diagnosis and relieve the condition. Gastric dilatation seldom occurs when a nasogastric tube has been inserted and is draining for the immediate postsurgical period. The condition can develop when a long intestinal tube is in the distal small bowel and ileus is present. The dangers of unrecognized acute gastric dilatation are those of fluid and electrolyte loss, perforation of the stomach, and aspiration pneumonitis.

FECAL IMPACTION

Postoperative fecal impaction may develop in a vigorous person as well as in the elderly postsurgical patient after a few days of bed rest. The common symptom is diarrhea and at times fecal incontinence. The patient has a constant sensation that the stool is not evacuated. The diagnosis is made by digital rectal examination. Manual disimpaction, which may need to be repeated several times, is the treatment. A rare and late event in fecal impaction is necrosis and perforation of the sigmoid.

POSTOPERATIVE PANCREATITIS

Acute pancreatitis following surgery is usually a result of upper abdominal surgery, particularly that of duodenal ulcer disease or biliary tract disease, but this may not always be the case. Postoperative pancreatitis carried a mortality twice as high as other types of pancreatitis seen at the Peter Bent Brigham Hospital.

The diagnosis is often obscure after major abdominal surgery. Any postoperative patient with unexplained volume deficit, renal failure, hypotension, and icterus in addition to upper abdominal pain must be evaluated for the possibility of pancreatitis. The amylase level is the best aid to the diagnosis, but it may not always be diagnostic since small bowel surgery *per se* may be associated with elevated levels of amylase. The same criteria that were mentioned for evaluating the serum amylase level in acute pancreatitis are operative (Chapter Twelve). Patients with previous pancreatitis are particularly susceptible and their disease is likely to be lethal.

When pancreatitis is associated with duodenal ulcer surgery and leakage of the duodenal turn-in develops, it is always essential to provide proper surgical drainage for the duodenum with a catheter duodenostomy if possible. Accurate replacement must be made of fluid and electrolyte losses, and the pancreas must be kept at rest until the process subsides. This is the only way in which the severe mortality of this condition can be appreciably reduced.

ACUTE POSTOPERATIVE CHOLECYSTITIS

Acute cholecystitis that develops in the postsurgical period after an operation for unrelated disease constitutes a surgical emergency. The *de novo* acute disease easily can be masked by the usual postoperative pain, slight temperature elevation, and ileus. Acute cholecystitis in the postoperative period occurs more frequently in males than females, more often in patients over 60 years of age, and has a higher percentage of acalculous cholecystitis than the usual instances of acute cholecystitis. Biliary stasis caused by postoperative fasting and the administration of narcotics is thought to be an important factor in the onset of acute postoperative cholecystitis. If the surgeon had the opportunity to palpate the gallbladder at the primary operation, he or she would be alerted to the possibility of the disease by the presence of biliary calculi. The diagnosis may be difficult and only an acute awareness of the potential for acute postoperative cholecystitis to develop permits prompt and proper treatment to be instituted, namely, cholecystectomy or cholecystostomy.

POSTOPERATIVE INTRAABDOMINAL ABSCESS

Abscess formation may occur after any abdominal operation, especially in situations in which there has been a perforation of a hollow viscus or the gastrointestinal tract has been opened. Classic examples of abscess formation are those that occur after perforated appendicitis and resections for regional enteritis and colonic diverticulitis. Complicating abscesses do not manifest themselves before 5 to 10 days, and the onset is insidious with rising temperature and increase in the pulse rate; chills and pain may or may not be a prominent part of the clinical picture. The evaluation of the abdomen may be clouded by residual incisional pain and some degree of paralytic ileus. Plain roentgenograms of the abdomen may provide a clue to the complication, but ultrasound scanning often will precisely define the location of the abscess (see Chapter Five). Once the abscess is diagnosed, it should be adequately drained with care not to spread purulent material into uncontaminated areas.

GLOVE STARCH PERITONITIS

Cornstarch (glove starch) peritonitis is an entity associated with the use of cornstarch as a surgical glove powder. It is postulated that the granulomatous lesion of the peritoneum is due to the reaction of the host to an inert foreign body or to a hypersensitivity to cornstarch. Clinical signs and symptoms develop, in most instances, 2 to 6 weeks postoperatively. The patient usually complains of malaise and may appear to be in a toxic condition. Some pyrexia, abdominal tenderness, paralytic ileus, and a palpable mass are other features that may be present. The diagnosis is difficult to make unless an abdominal tap is done and the aspirated fluid is examined microscopically with polarized light for the intracellular double refractile starch granules ("Maltese crosses"). Reoperation is not necessary if the diagnosis is known, since most patients seem to recover completely after a period of time. However, treatment with corticosteroids is effective in hastening the resolution of the lesion. The syndrome is not common when the numbers of laparotomies performed are considered.

PERFORATION DUE TO COLOSTOMY IRRIGATION

This seems to be an unlikely injury but it certainly occurs occasionally. It is one of the important reasons advanced by many surgeons for not having patients control their colostomies by irrigation. However, patients usually are carefully instructed in the technique of irrigating their colostomies, with emphasis on being gentle and never forcing the irrigating tube. The accident is more apt to happen when the patient uses a hard plastic catheter or a stiff, hard, rubber catheter. The diagnosis is usually apparent at once, since the patient feels immediate pain and shortly develops the signs of peritonitis. Most of the perforations are interperitoneal so that immediate operation is mandatory. Probably the best form of treatment is to dissect the stoma out and resect the area of perforation, since the perforations usually are not far away from the stoma itself. If there has been much fecal contamination drainage is recommended.

POSTOPERATIVE JAUNDICE

A mild degree of hyperbilirubinemia is probably a more frequent postoperative occurrence than realized. While clinical jaundice is much less common, it is of more serious portent and difficult to diagnose. Some causes of postoperative jaundice are listed in Table 18-1. In most instances mild elevations of the serum bilirubin level off in a few days and then decline. However, a steadily rising serum bilirubin is an indication of significant impairment of liver function. Occlusive trauma to

TABLE 18–1   Some Causes of Postoperative Jaundice

1. Hemolysis
2. Viral hepatitis
3. Drug or anesthetic toxicity
4. Septicemia
5. Liver hypoxia during operation
6. Leakage of bile into peritoneal cavity
7. Operative stress on preexisting liver disease
8. Pulmonary embolism
9. Retained common duct stone
10. Injury to the common bile duct
11. Pylephlebitis

the common bile duct results in immediate jaundice within a day or so, while infectious jaundice secondary to blood or blood products or a contaminated hypodermic needle has an incubation of over 5 weeks, and therefore usually does not develop until the patient has gone home. Reoperation, if indicated, is seldom necessary within 3 weeks for postoperative obstructive jaundice.

Some guidelines for the diagnostic approach to postoperative jaundice have been described by Morgenstern as follows:

1. Determine preoperative liver function when possible. The increased use of the automated blood chemistry profiles are helpful as they usually include bilirubin, alkaline phosphatase, and serum glutamic oxaloacetic transaminase determinations. Obviously if a subclinical hepatic dysfunction is known prior to operation, some effort can be made to protect the liver during the operation.

2. Review the anesthetic agents and all preoperative and postoperative medications to see if they are known to be icterogenic.

3. Serial liver function tests should be done, their chief value being to tell whether the jaundice is worsening or improving.

4. Look for sources of sepsis and make blood cultures.

5. Review the number of transfusions and check the age of the stored blood.

6. Rule out hemolysis or hemolytic syndromes.

7. Look for collections of sequestered blood.

8. Check renal function; it may be depressed in severely jaundiced patients.

9. Perform a liver biopsy during the operation if the liver does not appear normal. Routine liver biopsy does not seem justified in every upper abdominal operation. Liver biopsy in the immediate postoperative period does yield enough information to justify its use.

10. The color of the stool is of limited value in the differential diagnosis of intrahepatic and extrahepatic causes of jaundice, although a brown stool in the face of a rising serum bilirubin is suggestive of nonobstructive jaundice.

11. Retrograde fibroptic endoscopic cholangiography and percutaneous transhepatic cholangiography are techniques that are available for diagnosis of the cause of jaundice. In the postoperative jaundiced patient, these diagnostic tools are not used until the patient has recovered from his or her primary operation.

REFERENCES

Adams, T. W., and Foxley, G. F., Jr.: A diagnostic technique for acalculous cholecystitis. Surg. Gynecol. Obstet., *142*:168, 1976.

Anderson, W.: Boyd's Pathology for the Surgeon. 8th ed., Philadelphia and London, W. B. Saunders Co., 1967.

Ariel, I. M., and Kazarian, K. K.: Diagnosis and Treatment of Abdominal Abscesses. Baltimore, Williams & Wilkins Co., 1971.

Artz, C. P., and Hardy, J. D.: Complications in Surgery and Their Management. 3rd ed., Philadelphia, W. B. Saunders Co., 1975.

Baker, R. J., Toxman, P., and Freeork, R. J.: An assessment of the management of nonpenetrating liver injuries. Arch. Surg., *93*:84, 1966.

Botsford, T. W., Healey, S. J., and Veith, F.: Volvulus of the colon. Am. J. Surg., *114*:900, 1967.

Botsford, T. W., and Zollinger, R. M., Jr.: Diverticulitis of the colon. Surg. Gynecol. Obstet., *128*:1209, 1969.

Botsford, T. W., Zollinger, R. J., Jr., and Hicks, R.: Mortality of the surgical treatment of diverticulitis. Am. J. Surg., *121*:702, 1971.

Brewer, R. J., Golden, G. T., Hitch, D. C., Rudolf, L. E., and Wangensteen, S. L.: Abdominal pain: An analysis of 1000 consecutive cases in a university hospital emergency room. Am. J. Surg., *131*:219, 1976.

Brief, D. K., and Botsford, T. W.: Primary bleeding from the small intestine in adults. J.A.M.A., *184*:140, 1963.

Carlisle, B. B., and Lawler, M. R., Jr.: Aneurysm of the splenic artery. Am. J. Surg., *114*:443, 1967

Cope, Z.: The Early Diagnosis of the Acute Abdomen. London, Oxford University Press, 1972.

Cope, Z.: The growth of knowledge of acute abdominal diseases 1800–1900. Proc. R. Soc. Med., *57*:129, 1964.

Curtis, L. E., and Botsford, T. W.: Some pitfalls in the diagnosis of the acute abdomen. Med. Times, 1962 (Nov.).

Delaney, T., and Hoxworth, P. I.: Enteric-coated potassium chloride enteropathy. Surg. Gynecol. Obstet., *127*:76, 1968.

313

Dencker, H.: Pneumoscrotum as an early sign of anastomic leakage after anterior resection of the colon. Surg. Gynecol. Obstet., *134*:1005, 1972.

Dunphy, J. E., and Botsford, T. W.: Physical Examination of the Surgical Patient. 4th ed., Philadelphia and London, W. B. Saunders Co., 1975.

Dunphy, J. E., and Way, L. W.: Current Surgical Diagnosis and Treatment. 3rd ed., Los Altos, Calif., Lange Medical Publications, 1977.

Farha, G. J., and Robinson, F. W.: Mesenteric thrombosis. A diagnostic challenge. Am. J. Surg., *108*:47, 1964.

Haygood, F. D., and Polk, H. C., Jr.: Gunshot wounds of the colon. Am. J. Surg., *131*:213, 1976.

Haynes, C. D., Gunn, C. H., and Martin, J. D.: Colon injuries. Arch. Surg., *96*:944, 1968.

Holm, H. H., Kristensen, J. K., Rasmussen, S. N., Pedersen, J. F., and Hancke, S.: Abdominal Ultrasound. Munksgaard, Copenhagen, and Baltimore, University Park Press, 1976.

Jones, P. F.: Emergency Abdominal Surgery. Oxford, London, Edinburgh, Melbourne, Blackwell Scientific Publications, 1974.

Kaye, M. D.: Pleuropulmonary complications of pancreatitis. Thorax, *23*:271, 1968.

Knudson, R. J., and Zeiber, W. F.: Postoperative acute cholecystitis. N. Engl. J. Med., *269*:289, 1963.

Leopold, G. R., and Asher, W. M.: Fundamentals of Abdominal and Pelvic Ultrasonography (Vol. VI, Saunders Monographs in Clinical Radiology). Philadelphia, W. B. Saunders Co., 1975.

Madding, G. F., and Kennedy, P. A.: Trauma to the Liver (Vol. III, Major Problems in Clinical Surgery). 2nd ed., Philadelphia, W. B. Saunders Co., 1971.

McHardy, G., Bechtold, J. E., and McHardy, R. J.: Hemorrhage from primary disease of the mesenteric small intestine. Gastroenterology, *28*:17, 1955.

Moore, F. D.: Metabolic Care of the Surgical Patient. Philadelphia, W. B. Saunders Co., 1959.

Moore, H. D.: Diagnosis of rupture of abdominal aortic aneurysms. Lancet, *2*:184, 1967.

Moretz, W. H., and Erickson, W. G.: The diagnostic peritoneal tap. Am. Surgeon, *22*:1095, 1956.

Morgenstern, L.: Postoperative jaundice: An approach to a diagnostic dilemma. Am. J. Surg., *128*:255, 1974.

Moss, L. K., Schmidt, F. E., and Creech, O., Jr.: Analysis of 550 stab wounds of the abdomen. Am. Surgeon, *28*:483, 1962.

Nance, F. C., Wennar, M. H., Johnson, L. W., et al.: Surgical judgment in the management of penetrating wounds of the abdomen: Experience with 2212 patients. Ann. Surg., *179*:639, 1974.

Neck, W. V., Zollinger, R. W., and Pace, W. G.: Retroperitoneal hemorrhage after blunt abdominal trauma. J. Trauma, *7*:652, 1967.

Netterville, R. E., and Hardy, J. D.: Penetrating wounds of the abdomen; problems in management. Ann. Surg., *166*:232, 1976.

O'Connell, T. X., Kadell, B., and Tompkins, R. K.: Ischemia of the colon. Surg. Gynecol. Obstet., *142*:337, 1976.

Peterson, L. M., Collins, J. J., Jr., and Wilson, R. E.: Acute pancreatitis occurring after operation. Surg. Gynecol. Obstet., *127*:23, 1968.

Reuter, S. R., and Redman, H. C.: Gastrointestinal Angiography (Vol. 1, Saunders Monographs in Clinical Radiology). 2nd ed., Philadelphia, W. B. Saunders Co., 1977.

Romer, J. F., and Carey, L. C.: Pancreatitis: A clinical review. Am. J. Surg., *111*:795, 1966.

Root, H. D., Hauser, C. D., McKinley, C. R., et al.: Diagnostic peritoneal lavage. Surgery, *57*:633, 1965.

Sabiston, D. C., Jr.: Davis-Christopher Textbook of Surgery. 11th ed., Philadelphia, W. B. Saunders Co., 1977.

Samuel, E.: Gastrointestinal manifestations of vascular disease. Proc. R. Soc. Med., *60*:839, 1967.

Sugarbaker, P. H., et al.: Preoperative laparoscopy in diagnosis of acute abdominal pain. Lancet, Feb. 22:442, 1975.

Sugarbaker, P. H., McReynolds, R. A., and Brooks, J. R.: Glove starch granulomatous disease: An unsolved surgical problem. Am. J. Surg., *128*:3, 1974.

Sugarbaker, P. H., and Wilson, R. E.: Using celioscopy to determine stages of intra-abdominal malignant neoplasms. Arch. Surg., *111*:41, 1976.

Walters, R. L., Gaspard, D. J., and German, T. D.: Traumatic pancreatitis. Am. J. Surg., *111*:364, 1966.

Williams, L. F., Jr., Bosniak, M. A., Wittenberg, J., et al.: Ischemic colitis. Am. J. Surg., *117*:254, 1969.

Williams, L. F., and Byrne, J. J.: Trauma to the liver at the Boston City Hospital from 1955 to 1965. Am. J. Surg., *112*:368, 1966.

Worth, M. H., Jr.: Abdominal trauma. J.A.M.A., *235*:853, 1976.

Yoo, S. T., Vanecko, R. M., Freeork, R. J., and Shoemaker, W. C.: Unusual causes of the acute abdomen. Arch. Surg., *96*:296, 1968.

INDEX

Note: Page numbers in *italics* refer to illustrations. Page numbers followed by the letter "t" refer to tables.

317